Ochsner's

Ochsner's

AN INFORMAL HISTORY OF
THE SOUTH'S LARGEST PRIVATE
MEDICAL CENTER

John Wilds

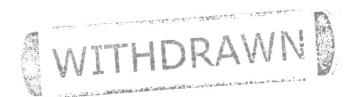

LOUISIANA STATE UNIVERSITY PRESS
BATON ROUGE AND LONDON

LIBRARY OF CONGRESS CATALOGING IN PUBLICATION DATA

Wilds, John.
Ochsner's: an informal history of the South's
largest private medical center.

Includes index.
1. Ochsner Medical Institutions—History. 2. Medical
Centers—Louisiana—New Orleans—History. I. Title.
RA982.N450388   1985   362.1′1′0976335   85′5779
ISBN 0-8071-1228-3

Contents

Illustrations

Preface

When Thomas P. Gore invited me in my retirement years to write a history of the Ochsner Medical Institutions, I went to work at once, while Alton Ochsner, Guy A. Caldwell, and Curtis H. Tyrone were still alive and Merrill O. Hines was beginning an assignment that would give him time to reminisce. Frank A. Riddick, Jr., and George H. Porter III were busy, but they ungrudgingly spared the hours for which I asked, as did Richard W. Freeman and J. Thomas Lewis. I had sources that no other chronicler ever again will be able to duplicate, along with free access to minutes, memoranda, correspondence, the written records of four decades of activity. I also referred continually to Dr. Caldwell's *Early History of the Ochsner Medical Center* (Springfield, Ill., 1965), a resource rich in facts.

The number of principals available for interviews is dwindling, and much of the source material is not part of the public record. Therefore, since the main purpose of footnote citations is to guide future researchers, they would be of doubtful value here, and I have not used them.

A strictly chronological account could have told of the planning, the inner conflicts, the changing environment, the triumph over adversity, all of which are factors in the evolution of the Ochsner Institutions. Such an approach might do justice to the story of a plow manufacturer or a department store. But here we are dealing with the elemental drama, man's struggle with death. The details of how a new hospital was financed belong in our narrative; even more so does the story of the surgeon who saved the life of a youth with a two-by-four stud driven all the way through his chest. On one level, we trace the development of a medical center that attracts more visitors to New Orleans every year than does Mardi Gras or the Sugar Bowl. On another level, we cite some of the reasons why the patients, many of them from Latin America, choose Ochsner. We recall medical breakthroughs, remarkable cases. We try to convey some of the excitement of the facility named for Alton Ochsner.

I have mentioned the names of a few of those who contributed so generously to the writing of this book. Dozens of others have been unstinting in their help—staff doctors, present and retired; administrators, old and new; nurses; secretaries; receptionists; patients. The list goes on and on, and specifically includes Elaine Ford, Rita Howard, Mary Knight, Carole Parks, and Karen Nabonne.

My debt to Merrill Hines is beyond payment. And finally, I acknowledge with deep appreciation the indispensable counsel and guidance of my wise and talented editor, Martha Lacy Hall, and the preparation of the manuscript by the most proficient of typists, Lynne Kuhlmann.

Ochsner's

Introduction

Never in medical history had pygopagus Siamese twins been success-fully separated. But when girls connected at the sacrum (the bottom of the spine) were born to the wife of the mayor of Lafayette, Louisiana, the attempt had to be made, for the alternative was death, or worse. And so, on Thursday morning, September 17, 1953, in an operating room at the Foundation Hospital, Alton Ochsner defied the odds. The chief of surgery of the Ochsner Clinic of New Orleans made an inci-sion in the skin over the place where the twins were joined, and then he went to work.

There was no gloom or feeling of impending failure among the doc-tors and nurses who ringed the table or peered over the shoulders of Ochsner and his assistants in this climactic scene of a drama that had begun at Lafayette nearly two months earlier. True, the literature cited only disastrous results, but perhaps no previous separation had been essayed by a surgeon as skilled as Alton Ochsner. Almost certainly, no surgeon had ever approached such a procedure with as much guidance and support as had been provided by the team of clinic practitioners who prepared the babies for their live-or-die ordeal.

Catherine and Carolyn were born, weighing a combined eleven pounds, eight ounces, on July 22 to Mr. and Mrs. Ashton J. Mouton. Two days later, when they were able to be moved, Mrs. Mouton's father, Henry Voorhies, a physician, sent them to the Foundation Hospital.

For one week general surgeons, neurosurgeons, internists, pediatri-cians, orthopedists, colon and rectal surgeons, neurologists, urologists, and radiologists probed to determine the extent to which nature had joined the tiny girls. The findings were encouraging. Each had her own separate vital organs. (Some Siamese twins are not so lucky.) The colons of both were connected to a single natural outlet, and their sacra were fused, but the problems appeared to be correctable.

On July 31 Dr. Ochsner performed preliminary surgery to provide a temporary colostomy—an outlet from the intestines—for each twin. By September 17 the girls were judged to be in condition for the surgical repairs intended to make possible a normal existence for each.

With deftness and economy of movement, the hallmarks of his operating technique, Ochsner carefully cut through the flesh until he exposed the sacrum. He found that the twins were united along the full measure of the bone and that their spinal canals were also joined. The challenge was to divide the sacrum and the canals without damaging the networks of nerves. One slip could result in paralysis. Ochsner's hand was as steady as it would inevitably prove in the twenty thousand operations of a long career. With scalpel, bone-cutting forceps, and scissors he made the twins individuals. Hospital records do not reveal how many glasses of cold tomato juice Ochsner consumed after this historic procedure, but it was a custom for nurses to have a plentiful supply chilled for him on his operating days.

As soon as the babies were parted, Carolyn was lifted to another table, and Rawley M. Penick, a general surgeon, began the tedious procedure of closing the surgical wounds of perhaps the tiniest patient he ever treated. Ochsner, meanwhile, was doing the same thing for Catherine. Two and a half hours after they were brought into the operating room, the twins were taken to separate cribs in the recovery room. Their vital signs were good, and although the job was not yet completed, Ochsner and his associates felt reasonably confident that they had won the gamble.

For years, Catherine and Carolyn were frequent patients at the Ochsner Medical Center. Plastic surgeons and gynecologists joined the other specialists in transforming two victims of a cruel natal anomaly into infants who in time would become normal, uncommonly pretty, and radiant young women. As babies and small children, they screamed when they saw the doctors who treated them most frequently—Ochsner, Merrill O. Hines, and Duncan McKee—but by the time they were in their teens, they would race to embrace the men whom they had come to see as benefactors.

The birth of Siamese twins is a rare phenomenon, and only 3 percent are of the pygopagus type. Fate dealt harshly with the Mouton girls, but that fickle lady relented when she picked the time and place. Had they been born a dozen years earlier, there would have been no institution in the Deep South where all the resources of medical science could have been marshaled in a single team able to separate them and help them grow into happy adulthood. But by 1953, only 150 miles east of Lafayette, a haven of hope had arisen, an association of surgeons and physicians that was taking its place alongside the Mayo Clinic, the Cleveland Clinic, the Lahey Clinic, and the Henry Ford Hospital as one of the premier group practices of America. The twins' grandfather, Dr. Voorhies, knew where he could turn for help without sending the infants on a risky journey to Rochester, Cleveland, Boston, or Detroit.

Five members of the Tulane University medical faculty had just such situations in mind on January 2, 1942, when they opened the doors to the Ochsner Clinic. They saw it as a medical court of last resort, a place to which practitioners could refer their difficult cases, a combination of talents that could be brought to bear on life-threatening problems—all this in a clinic where every diagnostic and therapeutic need could be filled in one building.

The concept of group—clinic—practice on a wholesale scale was slow to move into the Gulf South, and it was resisted by a medical community of traditional solo practitioners. But patients took to the idea of one-stop medical attention. By 1953 there were 150,448 patient appointments per year recorded at the Ochsner Clinic, a development that confirmed the fears of those who believed the group would take over an inordinate share of the diagnostic and therapeutic activity in New Orleans. The original clinic medical staff of nineteen had grown to seventy physicians and surgeons.

The twins were separated in the surgical area of a former army post hospital at Camp Plauché located in Jefferson Parish on the east bank of the Mississippi River alongside the Huey P. Long Bridge. It was a makeshift facility, utilized only because the need was pressing and nothing more suitable was available. In the next year, 1954, the prospering Ochsner Medical Institutions began moving all functions to the present multimillion dollar campus, also alongside the Mississippi, about two miles downstream from the original hospital.

In the new surroundings the Ochsner founders realized their dreams of a complex that would not only provide clinical care but also contribute to the advancement of medical knowledge through research projects and educational opportunities that would attract practicing physicians, graduate trainees, medical students, and technologists. Forty years after the clinic began, a staff of 184 physicians and surgeons and 210 training fellows was handling patient appointments at the rate of 280,000 each year. Nearly a tenth of the patients came from Central and South America. Almost one-half lived in Louisiana and other states of the Gulf South.

The group practice evolved into the biggest private health activity in Dixie. Under the banner of the Ochsner Medical Institutions, doctors treat sick people, a hospital provides beds and surgical facilities, scientists carry on extensive research centered on hypertension and breast cancer, young physicians and surgeons receive graduate training, schools are operated for medical technologists, practitioners take refresher courses, and a hotel provides food and lodging for patients and their families. But unlike medical schools with faculty clinics, where education has priority, or scientific institutes, where research is emphasized, the overriding purpose of the Ochsner Institutions remains patient care as the five founders intended.

Two separate legal entities mesh their operations on the Jefferson Highway campus as the components of the Ochsner Medical Institutions, which actually exist in title only. The older division of the institutions is the Ochsner Clinic; the other, organized in 1944, is the Alton Ochsner Medical Foundation. All of it is known to many Louisianians simply as Ochsner's.

The Ochsner Clinic comprises physicians and surgeons practicing forty-seven medical specialties and subspecialties. It is a partnership, owned and operated by the staff doctors. The clinic provides diagnoses and treatment on a professional, fee-for-service basis. It is self-supporting, never asking contributions from outside.

The Alton Ochsner Medical Foundation is a nonprofit corporation that operates the Ochsner Foundation Hospital, along with the research and educational programs. It also runs the Brent House hotel, restaurants, parking garage, health club, and other amenities for patients and public. Profits are devoted to the support of the investigative scientists, the educational programs, and the charitable services to patients who cannot pay. The foundation is dependent upon grants from the government and from private foundations and upon contributions from public-spirited individuals who are interested in the advancement of medicine.

Interlocking relationships bind clinic and foundation together. The foundation owns the campus and all the facilities on it. It is the landlord to the clinic, charging rent for the building that houses the doctors' offices and for the equipment. In turn, the clinic doctors make up the staff of the Ochsner Foundation Hospital. Very early, as will be recorded, the founders learned that they needed a foundation to assure perpetuation of the clinic and a hospital that would allow the clinic to thrive. During lean times, the clinic almost went broke itself in order to support the foundation. The bright, up-to-date buildings owned by the foundation would become empty ghost facilities were not thousands of patients attracted by the reputations of the clinic's specialists.

Laymen, businessmen of superior judgment, recognizing the promise of clinic and foundation, helped shape the destiny of both and continue to influence the activities of the foundation. Long after old age removed the last of the founders from the clinic's councils, a third generation of staff doctors makes the decisions about professional matters.

The figures bespeak financial success. An enterprise launched on an investment of less than $500,000—borrowed money—grew in four decades into an activity with an annual cash flow of more than $150 million. Facilities purchased for $101,000 metamorphosized into a campus now worth $200 million. A staff of nineteen practitioners, including consultants, multiplied into a corps of four hundred medical doctors, counting the fellows in training.

The founders rolled the dice and won. They went into debt to open a hospital, then built the present plant. They started training young doctors. They financed expensive research and educational programs. They overcame hostility in the professional community, prevailed over competition from rival practitioners and establishments. They survived a lean period of plunging revenues and had the wisdom to head off a revolt by bringing the staff into the ownership. Nothing came easily. They made the right decisions.

There is more to the Ochsner Medical Institutions than bricks and steel, CAT scanners and heart-lung machines, hefty payrolls exceeded by those of only a handful of industrial plants in the area, bustling lobbies and a small army of doctors, overflowing garage and parking lots, never-ending construction of added facilities. These are the tokens of achievement, and an account of how they came about is a part of the Ochsner story—but only a part. Told alone, that story misses the excitement of medical practice, of lives saved and lost, of surgical breakthroughs, of scientific discoveries, of exceptional men who had a dream. It misses the human side, and humanity is the rock on which the institutions were built.

While the builders were busy, so were the physicians and surgeons, giving succor to the suffering who came to the institutions as a last resort, flying off to other parts of the United States, to Europe, to South and Central America to reach those who could not make their way to New Orleans. Some of their achievements are recorded in the medical literature, others are written only in the grateful hearts of patients and those who hold them dear. These were deeds that lifted Ochsner out of the ordinary, and any account of the institutions' progress must not neglect them.

The Early Years

CHAPTER ONE

The Patients

The experiment was about to begin. Over the course of the next decades doctors would establish and create the South's largest private medical center. Always, they would make use of the most sophisticated techniques available and the most modern equipment. Often they would themselves create the techniques, invent the equipment. The doctors and the institutions they founded and operated would earn fame, would make their profit, would work out administrative squabbles to create a stable partnership that would stand the test of time. But while they were accomplishing these things, always before them would be the patient, the individual man, woman, or child who was sick and needed help. To aid one person, a new technique would be tried; out of failure to save another, a new piece of equipment would be invented. Such encounters produced the modern medicine that now can do so much to improve the lives of so many. The history of Ochsner is in large measure the story of how doctors got better and better at helping sick people.

A baby girl was born in a south Mississippi town on May 2, 1949, weighing eight and a half pounds and very sick indeed. Protruding from her mouth was a growth almost as large as her head. A tumor or a parasite, an undeveloped twin, it was known in medical terminology as an epignathus. Medical experience indicated the baby had no chance of survival; the literature contained no previous case in which the host lived.

Four and a half hours after her birth, the infant was admitted to the Foundation Hospital. The tiny girl, her airways largely blocked by the growth, was suffering acute respiratory distress. Within an hour, William B. Ayers performed a tracheotomy, slitting open her throat to insert a tube that facilitated breathing. For the first and perhaps only time of his life, he had to make a transverse incision because the neck was too short for the customary longitudinal opening. Only the inner lining of the smallest tracheotomy tube could be accommodated.

Respiration improved immediately, and Ayers turned to the next problem, providing nourishment. Because the tumor completely filled the mouth, the only recourse was a gastrostomy. Nineteen hours after birth, the surgeon operated again, to place a tube through the skin and into the stomach to allow direct feeding.

Four days after the birth, Alton Ochsner excised the growth, which extended far down into the pharynx. He had to sacrifice part of the hypertrophied tongue. At first the swollen tongue kept the baby from closing her mouth, and after closure of the gastrostomy she was fed her formula with a medicine dropper. Then the tongue receded, and she learned to suck the nipple of her bottle.

At the age of fourteen months, the girl weighed nineteen pounds. She could enunciate words clearly with a tongue that was almost normal in size and shape. Afterwards, when she was twelve years old, she entered the Ochsner Foundation Hospital twice for plastic surgery that repaired problems caused by scars remaining from the excision.

The outcome was a happy one for one of the smallest patients ever to undergo surgery at Foundation Hospital. And the literature—the September, 1951, issue of *Surgery*—recorded the first survival of the host of an epignathus.

Part of the prestige of the Ochsner Institutions derived from unprecedented success in such difficult cases, and part of it came from successful treatment of famous people. Three of the founders of the Ochsner Clinic paced the floor in an operating room at Touro Infirmary on June 12, 1946. Guy Caldwell, Edgar Burns, and Curtis Tyrone could not have concealed their anxiety if they had tried. No routine case had brought them together to watch as Dean Echols, the staff neurosurgeon, worked on the anesthetized patient on the table. Underneath the drapes lay the governor of Mississippi, Thomas L. Bailey. Echols' task, in a delicate procedure that would last for three hours, was to excise part of a giant follicular lymphoma and relieve intolerable pressure on the spinal canal. The outcome was in the balance, and so, to some extent, was the reputation of the Ochsner Clinic. No matter Echols' proficiency, if Bailey died the news stories would say he succumbed while undergoing surgery performed by an Ochsner staff doctor. There was bound to be a negative impact in Mississippi, whence came a good proportion of the young clinic's patients.

A month later Echols had a letter from the capitol at Jackson. "We can never voice or give expression to our gratitude for your faithful vigilance at a time when the *best* was needed in order for me to make the grade," Govenor Bailey wrote the surgeon. The operation served its purpose of relieving pain, but the progress of the cancer was inexorable, and in late November, the governor died. Mrs. Bailey wrote to Burns, who had shepherded her husband through earlier visits to the clinic: "You were more than a doctor to Thos. L. I shall always love you for going the second mile with us."

Bailey was the first of a series of Louisiana and Mississippi politicians to be treated by Ochsner practitioners. Governor Bailey had hardly gone home to recuperate from the Echols operation before Senator Theodore G. Bilbo of Mississippi appeared at the clinic with a carcinoma in the mouth. Alton Ochsner resected part of the mouth on August 31, 1946. In January, 1947, Bilbo entered the Foundation Hospital and underwent another operation. This time Ochsner removed part of the jawbone. The controversial politician, who lived at Poplarville, was back in the Foundation Hospital on August 7 and died there two weeks later of diffuse periarteritis nodosa.

The names of all but one of the Louisiana governors who have served since the clinic was opened appear on the Ochsner patient rolls. Sam H. Jones, the reform governor who rode into office in 1940 on the impetus of the Louisiana Scandals, was occasionally a clinic patient after he left office. Jimmie Davis was treated for stomach pains growing out of stress during his first term as Louisiana governor and occasionally saw Burns during his second term. Burns also prescribed for a kidney ailment that bothered Governor Robert F. Kennon during the latter's 1952–1956 term. Mrs. Kennon underwent gall bladder surgery at Foundation Hospital in 1953. Each night during her stay in the hospital the governor in Baton Rouge would call anesthesiologist Francis X.

LeTard, who had an apartment on the hospital grounds, for a detailed report on his wife's condition.

Earl K. Long's first visit to an Ochsner institution, the clinic, during his 1948–1952 term as governor was peaceful. He received X-ray treatment and physical therapy for pain in the shoulder resulting from an earlier coronary thrombosis. The Ochsner Foundation Hospital was thrown into turmoil, however, on June 17, 1959, when the governor entered during a frenzied interlude in which he was in and out of mental institutions and was fighting to prevent his ouster from office. Newsmen besieged the hospital during his overnight stay. The admission instructions denied him the use of the telephone and said: "Patient is never to be left alone, day or night, asleep or awake. Nurse will have to get replacement during her meals and ring for supplies not in patient's room."

Alton Ochsner had early experience dealing sensitively and discreetly with important political figures. One day during wartime, 1943, the telephone rang in his office at the Ochsner Clinic. On the line from Washington was Secretary of State Cordell Hull. He explained that Tomás Gabriel Duqué, the former president of the Republic of Panama, had done a favor for the United States by helping to defeat a pro-German government in his country. Now Duqué was critically ill of hyperthyroidism. Would Ochsner fly to Panama and try to save his life? The State Department would arrange the necessary airline priorities, Hull assured Ochsner.

On March 10, 1943, in the Santo Tomás Hospital, Ochsner performed a thyroidectomy. He stayed to see Duqué through a stormy recovery. The grateful newspaper publisher sent Ochsner a check for $10,000, the largest single fee of the surgeon's career.

Twelve years later Ochsner suspected that he was about to be involved in a cloak-and-dagger adventure when Edmundo Weiss, the Argentine air attaché in Washington, appeared uannounced at the clinic and asked to see him in the strictest privacy. Weiss, upon whom Ochsner had operated a few weeks earlier, described a fifty-nine-year-old man in Argentina who had begun having cramps in his left leg when he played tennis or walked fast. Did Ochsner think he could help the man? When Ochsner assured him that there were effective surgical procedures, Weiss revealed that the patient was Juan Domingo Perón, the president-dictator. In the political climate that existed in Argentina, it must not be known that Perón was having physical troubles. Weiss asked Ochsner to accompany him to Buenos Aires.

For the only time in all the years of his association, Ochsner arranged to leave the clinic without disclosing his destination to his associates. Mrs. Ochsner drove him to the New Orleans International Airport, where, suspense-story style, he was pointedly ignored by Weiss, who stood at a distance. Not until the Miami-bound plane was airborne did Weiss sit down beside Ochsner and fill him in on their travel plans. From Miami, they flew to Buenos Aires, where they were taken from the plane before it taxied to the terminal. Ochsner examined Perón in the seclusion of a presidential residence and determined that the president had peripheral artery disease involving the lower left leg. On January 25 in the residence, Ochsner successfully performed a novocaine sympathetic ganglion block in the area of the lumbar ganglia. Before leaving he also advised Perón to quit smoking.

Despite all precautions, a newspaper published by Argentine Socialist exiles in Montevideo, Uruguay, reported that Ochsner had gone to South America to see Perón and suggested that the president might have a tumor. Ochsner assured Perón that no information had emanated from New Orleans. In September the political ferment boiled over, and Perón had to flee Argentina. He went to Madrid, where Ochsner twice visited him in subsequent years. He found that Perón had followed the advice to give up cigarettes and, possibly as a result, required no further surgery.

Not all of the many thousands of Latin Americans treated by Ochsner doctors have been heads of state or wealthy men and women who could afford to fly to New Orleans for consultation or hospitalization. In 1975 a ten-year-old blind boy found begging on the streets of Tegucigalpa, Honduras, won the interest of a ham radio operator, who campaigned for money to get the lad to the clinic. Robert E. Schimek and William Williamson, donating their services, performed surgery that partially restored sight in the one eye that could be saved. In the 1950s Schimek, accompanied each time by an Ochsner fellow, made occasional trips, sometimes in Schimek's own plane, to a mission hospital at Santa Rosa in the Honduran mountains. There, working from dawn until midnight, they did eye operations for indigent patients who walked miles to reach the hospital when priests spread the word that the surgeons would be there. Later the construction of a highway enabled residents of the remote area to go to Honduran hospitals where ophthalmologists were available.

Forty years after the opening of the clinic, Latins accounted for some 28,000 patient appointments a year, 10 percent of the total. They made up a full 18 percent of the number of new patients. At first, most came from Central American countries, especially Guatemala and Nicaragua. But in the seventies the region was beset with political strife. Now, nearly three-fourths come from Venezuela, where prosperity built on oil production has resulted in the development of a sizable middle class that can afford foreign travel.

One day in August, 1981, sixty-two Venezuelans walked into the lobby of the clinic with longtime ties to their country and their continent. All of them expected to undergo medical checkups, but not one had a doctor's appointment. Most had purchased tours from travel agents who told them the packages included a visit to Ochsner.

Only the number in the party surprised receptionists and interpreters at clinic desks. Every Monday morning a score or two of Spanish-speaking visitors show up without making advance arrangements. They arrive the night before on the regular Sunday flight from Caracas. The influx puts a strain on schedules usually drawn up weeks in advance for nonemergency patients, but the tourists from afar are never turned away. They may have to wait for days, but all—even when there are sixty-two of them—get attention before returning home. A sampling of the numbers of Latin Americans who appeared without appointments in 1982 included 96 in January, 96 in February, 139 in March, 175 in April, 157 in May, and 132 in June.

The popularity of the clinic in Latin America is a legacy from Alton Ochsner. "When I came to Tulane in 1927," he recalled, "I found a number of Latin students enrolled in the medical school. I was attracted to them, and because I thought it important to cement the contacts, I cultivated them." Some of those whom he had taught returned home to practice medicine, and Ochsner began to receive invitations to make appearances in Central and South America. "I accepted as many as I could, and for some twenty years I spent a lot of time down there. After we started the Clinic, I proposed that I continue to go there. We had a tight budget, but I said this is no time to stint. I said I'd pay my own expenses if necessary. As a result we got Latin patients." Ochsner also recalled that one of the factors that induced the banker Rudolf S. Hecht to arrange the clinic's original financing was his knowledge that numerous Latin Americans came through New Orleans on their way to the Mayo, Cleveland, and Lahey clinics. "Mr. Hecht said they would stay in New Orleans for treatment if they knew there was a good clinic here," said Ochsner. Willoughby E. Kittredge said, "The Latins discovered us. They learned that they didn't have to go to Cleveland or Minnesota. They found out they didn't even have to bring winter clothes with them."

There are many reasons why Latin Americans choose to come to the United States for treatment. Although many South American doctors are capable practitioners, South American hospitals and clinics generally do not have diagnostic and therapeutic equipment as sophisticated as that found in up-to-date institutions in this country. Moreover, fees in the Central and South American areas are high, and often a patient can pay his airfare and hotel bills and still save money by coming to the United States for treatment.

The reasons so many Latin Americans choose Ochsner over institutions in Houston and Miami have to do with Alton Ochsner's fame, of course, and also with his legacy of outreach. The location of the Brent House hotel and restaurants on the campus makes it easy for Latin Americans to follow their custom of bringing their families with them when they visit the clinic or hospital. The size of a Latin's entourage is said to be a dependable indicator of his personal wealth. And Ochsner maintains a staff of about thirty-five interpreters who are available not only to guide Spanish-speaking patients through the routine of making and meeting appointments but also to translate the dialogue between doctor and patient.

Translating the language is important, but the interpreters must also translate two distinct and very different cultures to each other. Aminta Alfaro, who was born in Nicaragua, went to work as the third Ochsner interpreter in 1945. From the first, she related, Latin Americans have shown up without appointments. "We've always finagled a way to take care of them. Time has no meaning for them. They come at their own convenience and realize they will have to wait to see a doctor. They're almost all reasonable about delays, and they go away happy with the service." Vickie Garsaud now supervises the interpreters who make arrangements for non-English-speaking patients. The interpreters know at all times where to find those who are waiting, and doctors cooperate if they have a cancellation by giving the time to one of the walk-ins.

The staff has also attempted to nurture friendships formed by Alton Ochsner with Latin American physicians. Invitations to Ochsner doctors to participate in medical meetings or to lecture down below bring quick acceptance. Spanish-speaking staff members, among them the late C. Harrison Snyder and Mary Sherman and more recently gynecologist George T. Schneider, have been in demand.

Some travel agents have approached Ochsner with deals in which they would offer checkups at the clinic as part of prepaid tours. The administrative director Francis F. Manning has turned them down because the clinic does not want third parties to intervene between doctors and patients. In any case, Latin Americans are only part of an army of outsiders who are drawn to New Orleans because of the reputation of the Ochsner Institutions. Figures show that the annual influx exceeds the numbers of out-of-towners attracted by the Sugar Bowl football game, or even the Super Bowl. The impact on the economy of the metropolitan area is considerable, as Mayor de Lesseps S. Morrison recognized when he reacted with concern in 1950 to a rumor that the clinic might move to Houston.

The impact of Ochsner on the world's medicine is also significant. Not only do the new techniques and equipment developed at Ochsner eventually change medical practice in countries far from home, but the patients continue to come from far away and Ochsner doctors continue to travel. W. Larimer Mellon, Jr., who served as a fellow in general surgery at Ochsner in 1955, later established and operated a hospital for destitute natives in rural Haiti. The member of the financier Pittsburgh family was inspired by the example of Albert Schweitzer's hospital in Africa for the treatment of people who otherwise would have been without medical care. Ochsner doctors have gone to Haiti on occasion to help in Mellon's hospital.

Alton Ochsner went traveling again in 1949. On February 22 Ben Hogan had been seriously injured near Van Horn, Texas, in a collision between his automobile and a bus. Taken to an El Paso hospital, he had begun recovery from his injuries when blood clots developed in his veins. The thromboses caused collapse of one lung and would have been fatal had they reached the heart.

Physicians gave anticoagulants to try to halt the formation of clots and summoned Alton Ochsner from New Orleans. He was given a ride to El Paso on a B29 bomber. Seated in the bombardier's station in the nose of the plane, Ochsner noted furious activity on the airport below as the pilot circled for a landing. Ambulances and fire trucks were converging near a runway. Only after he was on the ground did the surgeon learn that the stir was caused by the B29. Lights on the instrument panel had indicated trouble with the landing gear, and the ground crew had been preparing for a crash that turned out to be a false alarm.

At the hospital, Ochsner determined that the only way to be sure the clots would not reach Hogan's heart would be to tie off the vena cava, the main vein. Hogan's wife, Valerie, objected. Somebody had told her that the procedure would cripple the patient's legs, and she did not want the responsibility for a decision that might prevent Hogan from playing golf again. The confident Ochsner met the issue head on. He promised her that her husband would be able to play.

After restoring the clotting mechanism so that Hogan would not bleed to death during surgery, Ochsner carried out the ligation. The patient's recovery was rapid. Within weeks he was practicing his swing again, and he want on to some of his greatest triumphs. Six of his nine major titles were won after the accident, and Ochsner's skills were reflected in golf's record books.

Tears glistened in Ben Hogan's eyes on the night in 1950 when he made a speech at a banquet at the Roosevelt Hotel opening a campaign for funds to build the Ochsner Foundation Hospital. "I know what Dr. Ochsner did for me," the golf champion said, explaining a rare show of emotion by a man noted on the links for his cool, poker-faced play. Hogan's gratitude moved him to accept the chairmanship of the fund-raising drive.

In later years he occasionally returned to the hospital that he had helped to make possible for treatment of bone and muscle ailments resulting from the injuries received in the accident. In 1957 while Hogan was still competing on the professional tour, he visited the clinic because of shoulder pain that became acute whenever he practiced for a tournament. Harry D. Morris prescribed conservative treatment. Again in 1962 Morris outlined remedial exercises to ease shoulder pain. In 1963, 1968, and 1969 Hogan underwent shoulder surgery, once performed by Morris and twice by A. William Dunn.

Hogan's faith in the Ochsner Institutions led to an interval in the Foundation Hospital that had the nurses atwitter and later sent Alton Ochsner winging off to Paris to perform an operation in unfamiliar surroundings. The motion picture star Gary Cooper, scheduled to begin filming the classic western *High Noon*, found himself incapacitated by a right inguinal hernia. Two previous operations had failed to bring lasting relief. Hogan learned of his friend's plight and advised him to seek Ochsner's surgical services. On March 13, 1952, Cooper arrived at Splinter Village, sending patients and personnel scurrying through the corridors for a glimpse. The next day Alton Ochsner repaired the hernia, and Cooper was able to complete the movie on schedule.

Seventeen months later Cooper was in Paris when he discovered he had a hernia on the left side. Because of income tax regulations, the star could not return to the United States before the end of the year. Again he called on Alton Ochsner. Accompanied by his wife, the surgeon took a sleeper plane to Paris, and on August 14, 1953, repaired the hernia in the American Hospital. In 1957 Cooper was a houseguest of the Ochsner's over Mardi Gras while he underwent a checkup at the clinic. There was no sign then of the cancers that led to his death in Hollywood on May 13, 1961.

The celebrities who come to Ochsner provide a special kind of excitement that people find hard to resist. But most of the patients who come to the medical institutions are known only to their own small circle of family and friends. Because Ochsner exists, such people can and do receive care as fine as any given the richest, most famous people on earth.

A receptionist halted ambulance attendants who were rolling a stretcher into the Foundation Hospital late on the afternoon of Thursday, November 18, 1948. "Wait. He'll have to sign a release," she said, indicating the sheet-covered figure on the stretcher. "Ma'am, he can't sign anything," said the attendant as he pulled back the sheet. The receptionist took one horrified look and fainted.

There lay twenty-one-year-old Dwight L. Lott of Poplarville, Mississippi. Out of his chest protruded one end of a two-by-four stud and out of his back jutted the other end. Four hours earlier an automobile in which Lott was a passenger went out of control and rammed a bridge near Bogalusa. A bridge railing penetrated the front of the car, jammed all the way through Lott's torso and tore into the rear of the vehicle. Rescuers had to saw the timber in two places in order to release the impaled passenger.

Lott regained consciousness while he was being freed. He was taken to a Bogalusa hospital, where a physician made a quick decision. "There's nothing I can do here," he said. "There's only one place I know of where they might be able to help you. That's the Foundation Hospital."

Alerted that an accident victim was enroute, Champ Lyons was scrubbed and waiting in the operating theater. He made an incision around the patient's side, connecting the wounds of entrance and exit. Two fractured ribs were divided to expose the ten-inch length of lumber, which Lyons lifted out. He found that it had missed the heart but lacerated a lung lobe, the diaphragm, and the spleen. The stomach had herniated into the chest. Dr. Lyons excised the spleen, repaired the torn tissues, closed the chest wall, and administered tetanus toxoid. Fifteen days later the rapidly convalescing Lott was transferred to the Veterans Administration Hospital at Biloxi, Mississippi.

Three decades afterward, Lott was in good health, living in Poplarville, and working in the construction business. Except for faded surgical scars, he had nothing more to remind him of his brush with death than a blurry snapshot to show that a man with a two-by-four-inch hole all the way through his chest would live.

CHAPTER TWO

Establishing the Clinic

The April 9, 1927, issue of the *Journal of the American Medical Association* explained the origins of the term *clinic*. The Greek *klinein* meant to lie down or recline. In its nominative form, *klinē*, it signified a bed. Gradually, the word took on the meaning of a bed of sickness and then practical instruction at the bedside. Thus, the French word *clinique* was used for an institution at which bedside teaching was emphasized, and in the United States, too, *clinic* was first applied to a teaching institution. Finally, doctors began to call their group practices clinics, as *JAMA* said, "perhaps by the want of a better term, perhaps for the purpose of conveying to the public the idea of greater importance or of institutional dignity." By 1939 the AMA judicial council was commenting that the term "now in the lay mind implies a very superior service by very superior individuals, which too frequently is not the case."

Many of the early groups were family enterprises; the Mayo brothers organized the first of the superclinics in 1907. In 1922 the AMA could identify only 139 clinics in the United States; by 1932 there were 270 listed; and in 1941 the number stood at 335. Of this number, one-third had only 3 physician members, and more than half counted 4 or fewer. The average was 6.2 members.

A study by the AMA published by the *Journal* on July 12, 1941, noted that group medicine had been influenced by the frontier phase of scientific medicine. More clinics than ever before appeared between 1919 and 1923. "This was the time when the scientific discoveries of Pasteur, Lister, Koch, and the Curies were firing the new generation of physicians with enthusiasm for laboratory methods." The young doctors went out to practice where laboratories and hospitals were scarce or even nonexistent. "It is natural that they joined into groups where some of the members could give 'special attention' to the phases of medicine in which they were most interested. Their pooled funds made possible some sort of a laboratory and often of a hospital." World War I took many doctors away from their regular practices "and accustomed them to work under military discipline where they were supplied facilities not available in many sections of the country. When these physicians returned they found in many cases that their practices had disappeared, and they sought a new start by associating in groups." Along with pioneer medicine and the lessons of World War I, the AMA *Journal* cited the spectacular success of the Mayo Clinic as providing impetus for the spread of clinics. In 1941 twelve states with only one-third of the nation's population boasted two-thirds of the clinics in operation. They were Texas, Wisconsin, Minnesota, California, Kansas, Oklahoma, Indiana, Illinois, Iowa, Nebraska, North Dakota, and Michigan.

Yet despite growing popularity, in the early 1940s the clinic was still an uncommon enterprise. Most cities—and certainly New Orleans— were citadels of traditional practice garrisoned almost entirely by solo practitioners. The idea of establishing a clinic in a city like New Orleans was a farsighted one indeed, and it was fully vindicated. Nowadays the AMA defines *group medical practice* as "the application of medical services by three or more physicians formally organized to provide medical care, consultation, diagnosis, and/or treatment through the joint use of equipment and personnel, and with the income from medical practice distributed in accordance with methods previously determined by members of the group." By 1965 the AMA identified 4,289 such groups, and the proliferation was barely begun. By 1969 the number was 7,891; by 1975 it was 8,483; and in 1980 the list had grown to 10,762. In a 1980 survey the AMA determined that 88,290 physicians—one fourth of all the doctors in the United States not employed by the federal government—were affiliated with groups. By far most of the group physicians—54,122, or 61.3 percent—were members of multispecialty clinics. Single-specialty groups accounted for 29,456 physicians (33.4 percent), and 4,712 (5.3 percent) worked in family practice clinics. By that time the Ochsner clinic had become one of the titans.

Nobody can say exactly when the first serious idea originated for a clinic made up of teachers at the Tulane University School of Medicine. Alton Ochsner had come to Tulane as chairman of surgery in 1927. Years later he recalled his early realization that the New Orleans medical community was attracting too few patients from the South, where progress in medical practice lagged behind the rest of the country, and from Latin America. Latins, he noted, were landing at New Orleans and immediately moving on to one of the big-name clinics in the North or East.

By 1938, when Guy A. Caldwell came to New Orleans as professor of orthopedics at Tulane, Ochsner had become perhaps the most influential practitioner in New Orleans. His national reputation surpassed that of any other New Orleans surgeon of his generation. Caldwell, a believer in the clinic philosophy, was interested in joining other New Orleans specialists in a group practice. He quickly realized that Alton Ochsner, because of his prominence at Tulane and his get-it-done personality, would be the key to any successful clinic in the area. One day, in a drugstore across the street from Touro Infirmary, Caldwell encountered Dean H. Echols, a neurosurgeon who had an office near Ochsner's at Tulane and frequently chatted with him. Caldwell asked him if he thought Ochsner would be interested in forming a group practice. Echols, remembering conversations with Ochsner, replied, "I know he would."

The event that actually set the wheels turning toward the creation of the Ochsner Clinic was the visit to Tulane in early 1940 of Dr. John Lockwood. Lockwood, a professor at the University of Pennsylvania Medical School, spoke enthusiastically of plans by some of the Pennsylvania faculty to organize a group practice, and he found a receptive audience. After Lockwood's visit, Ochsner sounded out several of his fellow faculty members at Tulane, including Caldwell; Francis E. Le-Jeune, otolaryngologist; and Edgar Burns, urologist. Finding the three physicians receptive, Ochsner broached the idea of a clinic at Tulane to Esmond Phelps, president of the board of administrators of the Tulane Educational Fund, and C. C. Bass, dean of the medical school. "Both of these gentlemen discouraged the plan," Caldwell recorded, "because they believed it would create discord and jealousy among the faculty members who would not be included in the group, and probably would be criticized by the school's alumni in the surrounding area." If there had been any hope that a new clinic could be launched in a friendly climate, the administrators' reaction dispelled it, but Ochsner and the other doctors were undeterred. Convinced they had a workable enterprise in mind, they continued their planning. This was only the first of many unsuccessful overtures toward a merger with Tulane.

On a Sunday morning in the spring of 1940, Curtis H. Tyrone, Tulane gynecologist and obstetrician, met with Ochsner, Burns, LeJeune, and Caldwell at Ochsner's home on Exposition Boulevard. They decided to explore the possibility of establishing a private clinic, most members of which would be on the Tulane faculty but which would be an entity separate from the university and medical school. It was an idea that would eventually create profound changes in the availability of health care in New Orleans, but almost two years would pass before the planning begun that morning would reach fruition.

The Tulanians envisioned a tertiary care unit in which specialists from all the medical disciplines would work together to diagnose and treat serious illnesses that overtaxed the capabilities of primary care physicians. Certainly, referral to specialists was nothing new. Under the procedure then current and still prevalent, a primary care physician would send a patient with appendicitis to a surgeon, or one with a kidney ailment to a urologist or one with a mental problem to a psychiatrist. If a patient's symptoms were baffling, he might be routed to three or four specialists, all in different parts of the city, much like the housewife who bought meat at the butcher shop, bread at the bakery, fish at the market, and vegetables at a stand across town.

The clinic was to serve as a medical supermarket. In one building would be assembled a corps of specialists who would work together to take care of patients referred by outside physicians or attracted by the clinic's reputation for excellence. The clinic would be geared toward patients who needed the attention of specialists—the seriously ill—but the founders foresaw that a demand for primary care would also have to be met.

The five founders were confident of their abilities, but they recognized the need for a strong department of medicine, an important element in any group. They approached Dr. John Herr Musser, professor of medicine at Tulane. However, Musser was reluctant, because of his hypertension, to commit himself to a busy work schedule. He declined the invitation to join the group as a founding member but agreed to join the staff as a consultant in internal medicine. The founding members next approached Dr. James Harold Watkins, a protégé of Dr. Musser's who had left the Tulane faculty in 1930 to establish a practice in internal medicine at Montgomery, Alabama, but maintained a close friendship with Alton Ochsner and Curtis Tyrone. He so seriously considered returning to New Orleans to join in the project that his name was included on an early application for a bank loan, but he finally concluded that he did not want to give up the independence of his practice and accept a reduction of income. During the remainder of his life he referred many patients to the clinic, however, and his eldest son, J. H. Watkins, Jr., was on the Ochsner staff for three years.

Despite the difficulty in obtaining a fine internist to head the department of medicine, the founders began making concrete efforts toward their goal. Ochsner returned to Phelps and Bass to propose that the five professors be retained on the Tulane faculty while they operated their own independent clinic. Bass offered no objection, and Phelps was enthusiastic. "Good," he told Ochsner. "We can have our cake and eat it, too." He did caution against shoving off on an ambitious enterprise when it was becoming apparent that the United States might soon be involved in a war.

The five professors found more encouragement at the 1940 meeting of the Southern Surgical Association in Hot Springs, Virginia. Frank H. Lahey, founder of the Lahey Clinic in Boston, and surgeons affiliated with the Mayo and Cleveland clinics agreed that New Orleans was a promising site and that the five Tulanians were well qualified to operate a clinic if they would enlist an outstanding internist on the staff. Lahey offered some advice that the founders would not forget. He told them to keep the power in a few hands; he alone, he said, made all major decisions at his clinic. He warned them to obtain an office building that would permit rapid expansion and not to try to operate a hospital. They should send patients to existing facilities. Finally, he advised them to resign their medical school appointments in order to work full-time for the clinic.

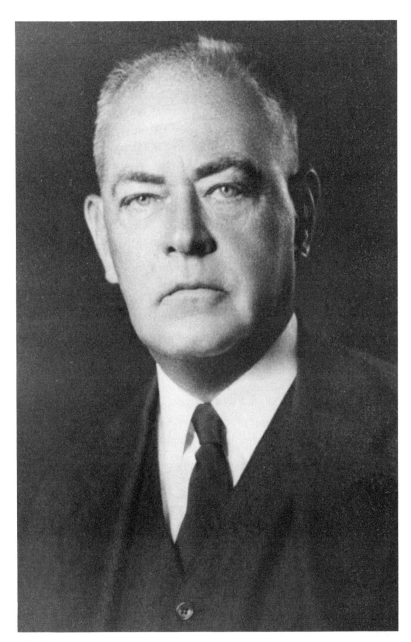

John H. Musser

Later that year, Alton Ochsner sought more of Lahey's advice, worrying about the advisability of going deep into debt to form the clinic. On November 5, 1940, Lahey replied that he would like to help Ochsner make a decision, but he added, "I cannot do that because I cannot take the responsibility of getting you involved financially. . . . I do not need to tell you that the ideal way to practice any branch of medicine is in a clinic where you can take everybody in regardless of their situation and make the costs fit their circumstances, where you can have the combined efforts of a variety of minds and interests, where you can improve your knowledge constantly by the contact with men in other fields." And he repeated his admonition about strong leadership. "Every clinic I have seen succeed has been dominated—perhaps directed is a better word—by an individual on whom rests ultimate responsibility. The most important thing is who would dominate the situation—does he have business judgment and experience to handle finances, and how much money would you personally have to put in and risk? I hope you go slow in committing yourself and Isabel [Mrs. Ochsner] in anything that involves you financially. It will be fine if it goes, but bad if you lose money." Ochsner's concern is understandable when his financial situation is remembered. He was paid only $10,000 a year as chairman of surgery at Tulane, and he picked up some additional income from private practice, but now he was to assume a share of debt running into hundreds of thousands of dollars.

The five professors believed their individual practices would bring in enough patients to send the clinic off to a fast start. They decided early on to avoid disputes over money by dividing the net income of the clinic, and the liabilities, equally. But even though all were successful practitioners, their combined savings fell far short of the kind of money needed to start the clinic. A building would have to be purchased or rented, furnished, and equipped. A laboratory was obviously essential. Staff physicians and surgeons would have to be hired, as would nurses, technicians, receptionists, and maids, and until collections began to trickle in, the salaries of all these people would be a drain on the capital. Thus, preliminary discussions focused on fund-raising ideas.

The organizers first sought capital from foundations and from local philanthropists, but nobody in New Orleans was interested in funding a private clinic. Nor were the banks eager to lend them money. The

Tulane physicians, all professionally and socially prominent and all members of the exclusive clubs of the city, got sympathetic hearings from their financier friends, but when the magnitude of their project, compared with their resources, was brought out, the risks became apparent. LeJeune did get a pledge of support from A. P. Imahorn, president of the Hibernia National Bank, but the most important development should be credited to Caldwell. One of his patients was Mrs. Rudolf S. Hecht, who was confined to a wheelchair as the result of an orthopedic ailment. On one of his visits to Mrs. Hecht, Caldwell discussed the plans for a clinic with her husband, chairman of the board of the Hibernia National Bank, chairman of the Mississippi Shipping Company, and one of the founders of the International Trade Mart, a civic project devoted to the development of New Orleans as a world trade center. When Rudolf Hecht responded favorably to the notion, Caldwell arranged a luncheon meeting with Ochsner.

"We told him we thought a clinic would attract people to New Orleans, and most particularly would bring in patients from Latin America," Ochsner recalled. "We explained that we had no collateral. He said he thought it would be a good thing for the city, and he arranged to lend us up to half a million dollars on our signatures." Hecht thus became the first of a small group of businessmen and lawyers who dedicated themselves to the development of the Ochsner Institutions and whose guidance enabled the medical men to avoid fiscal pitfalls and to operate an efficient enterprise, a suitable environment for their healing activities. He directed Ochsner and Caldwell to obtain an option on a suitable site for the clinic, to get estimates on the cost of erecting a building, and to apply to the board of directors of his bank for a loan.

Stanley M. Lemarie, a real estate agent, was enlisted to search for a location near Touro Infirmary, where all five surgeons admitted most of their private patients. Lemarie's first hope was the Otto F. Briede property, former residence of Dr. Henry Newman, at St. Charles Avenue and Foucher Street, a block from Touro. Lemarie conveyed an offer of $70,000 against the owner's asking price of $80,000. Because the property was in a residential area, however, a zoning change was required if it were to be used for a medical facility. Seventy percent of the landowners in the neighborhood agreed to such a change with their signatures on a petition. But the clinic met its first public opposition from

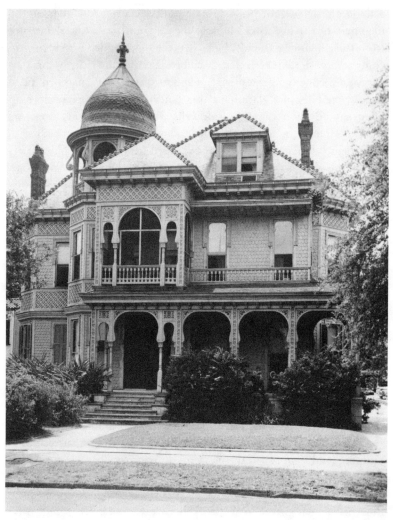

The old Briede home fronting on St. Charles Avenue, where ambulatory patients of the clinic resided some area residents headed by John E. Jackson, Louisiana's Republican party national committeeman, who contended the clinic would be a neighborhood nuisance. The controversy was just beginning.

So far, the efforts to organize the group had been made behind the scenes, but the application for the zoning change brought the first publicity. "Physicians ponder 'Little Mayo Clinic' for New Orleans," said a New Orleans *Item* headline on December 4, 1940. The news story told of plans for a clinic "where people from all over the South and from South and Central American countries could come for diagnostic checkups by groups of the most skilled medical specialists in the city." Ochsner was the only doctor named. In an editorial two days later the *Item* said the clinic should be encouraged by the public. "Dr. Ochsner's standing in the medical profession at large ought to be a guarantee that he and his associates will maintain standards that will make their enterprise a real public utility. It ought also to bring still more persons to New Orleans for the service that such institutions provide." The *Times-Picayune* also endorsed the proposed clinic. At a public hearing, the doctors' attorney, J. Blanc Monroe, pointed to the benefits that would accrue from the facility, citing the success of the Mayo and Johns Hopkins clinics. He promised that the building would not be turned into a hospital, as Jackson had suggested. The New Orleans Commission Council finally approved the rezoning, but by that time the Ochsner five had decided not to proceed in the face of the remaining opposition of some neighbors.

Lemarie looked elsewhere and discovered an even more desirable prospect, the five-story Physicians and Surgeons Building at Prytania and Aline streets, directly across Prytania from what was then the Touro entrance. It was in the most distinguished medical neighborhood in New Orleans, the first concentration of doctors' offices to develop as a satellite of a hospital. At the time, two-thirds of the city's practitioners rented offices in the central business district. Forty years later only one-fifth of the medical community was headquartered downtown, most doctors having moved to office complexes that had grown up around the hospitals. The Touro area in 1940 was a hub of distinguished medical practice. Next door to the Physicians and Surgeons Building on the Prytania Street side was the former office and home of the late E. Denegre Martin, an influential surgeon throughout the first third of the twentieth century. On the Aline Street side was the office of Isidore Cohn, the biographer of Rudolph Matas, New Orleans' internationally famous physician, whose own office was at 3521 Prytania Street. On the ground floor of the Physicians and Surgeons Building was a pharmacy, and twenty-five practitioners had offices there. The building had more space than the founders expected to need at the start, but heeding Lahey's advice to think big, they also made offers for the Martin site on Prytania and the Atwood Rice home two doors away on Aline.

By the time the plans for a clinic became public knowledge, the New Orleans medical community was seething—and no wonder. Every one of the five founders would have made anybody's list of the ten most successful practitioners in New Orleans. Moreover, Thomas Findley would head the internal medicine section and Matas and Musser would come in as part-time consultants. The group had also taken on a young thoracic surgeon, an associate of Ochsner's, who was only beginning to come into his own but who was already recognized as having rare gifts in the operating room. The young surgeon would later move to Houston where he would win worldwide acclaim rivaling that of Ochsner himself. He was Michael E. DeBakey. An all-star team was about to play under the Ochsner banner. All of the other storied clinics in the United States orbited around a single great figure or, in the case of the Mayo Clinic, two stars. But here, competing for patients with every practitioner in the city, a group was starting with more talent than any other clinic had ever assembled for a beginning.

The resentment boiled over in New Orleans on the night of Holy Thursday, April 13, 1941, when a messenger delivered to the home of each founder a small leather sack containing thirty silver dimes and a typewritten note: "To help pay for your Clinic. From the Physicians, Surgeons and Dentists of New Orleans." None of the five felt like Judas Iscariot, but all were stung by the rebuke from their colleagues. "I had friends who never spoke to me again," Tyrone recalled. Mrs. LeJeune received a telephone call telling her to "try to talk Duke [Dr. LeJeune] out of making a mistake. Don't let him get mixed up with that clinic." Willoughby E. Kittredge, who joined the urology department at the start, was given the cold shoulder by his college roommate.

New Orleans practitioners were not the only ones to attack the prin-

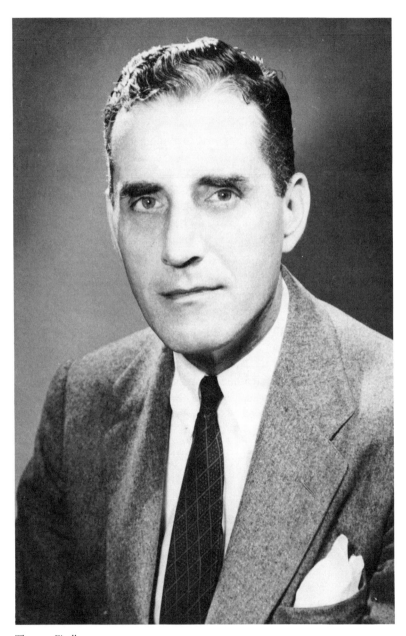

Thomas Findley

ciple of group medicine, but by the time Ochsner was getting started, the issue had already been settled by the American Medical Association, the profession's supreme arbiter in matters of morals and ethics. The AMA was told at its convention in 1941 that a search through the past thirty-two years of proceedings of the House of Delegates "failed to show any action that indicated the slightest hostility to the formation of ethical and capable medical groups." In 1933 the House of Delegates had commented, "Those forming a group should be guided by the same principles regarding professional qualifications for practice, ethical relations to fellow practitioners and consideration for the economic position of those whom they serve as should guide the individual practitioner." And later, in 1957, the house affirmed that "it is within the limits of ethical propriety for physicians to join together as partnerships, associations or other lawful groups provided that the ownership and management of the affairs thereof remain in the hands of licensed physicians."

The founders were not without friends in their profession. A few practitioners sensed the possibilities, and were eager to join in the clinic from the beginning. The two who showed the most interest were Neal Owens and Dean H. Echols, young men who shared space in the office of John Pratt in the American Bank Building. Owens went on to establish himself as the leading plastic surgeon of his time in New Orleans. Echols, a pioneer in spinal disc operations, won national standing in the field of neurological surgery. Owens suggested to Echols that they offer to become partners, but Echols felt that neither had the funds to finance their shares. Owens brushed aside the objection, pointing out they could borrow the money. In the summer or fall of 1941 the two met Caldwell and one or two of the other professors on the sidewalk outside Touro Infirmary and asked to be included. Caldwell explained that Blanc Monroe considered the partnership too large already and had advised against expanding it. Caldwell was willing, however, to include both doctors on the starting staff as consultants and to hire them full-time as soon as the volume of patients warranted it. Thus the names of Echols and Owens appeared on the original clinic letterhead. Owens was invited a few months later to take a place on the regular staff, but he declined and continued independent practice. When Caldwell telephoned Echols in May, 1942, and told him the time had come, Echols did not even ask what his salary would be. He did not discover until his first payday that he would be paid $10,000 a year. From the first day, he had an office on the fifth floor of the clinic building, next to Ochsner's. In the years to come Echols' influence earned him the right to be considered the sixth founder.

Among the decisions to be made in establishing the clinic was selecting a name. Ochsner suggested New Orleans Clinic or Southern Clinic, neither of which appealed to the others. They waited until Ochsner was in Ogden, Utah, for a meeting, then agreed among themselves. "The baby has a name. The Ochsner Clinic," they informed the surgeon in a telegram. Later Caldwell revealed that there was never any real question. "The Mayo, Lahey and other clinics each had the name of its chief surgeon. He's the one who had the drawing power. He carried the weight. And as we told each other, no matter what we named it people were going to call it the Ochsner Clinic. So we went ahead and named it Ochsner and were done with it."

The organization took legal form on May 2, 1941, in the office of the attorney J. Blanc Monroe in the Whitney Bank Building. Two entities were established. The Ochsner Clinic Associates became a partnership for the group practice of medicine. The Ochsner Clinic, Inc., was incorporated as a property-owning business. Under terms of the arrangement worked out by Monroe, the associates were to lease offices, laboratories, and other facilities from the corporation. Ochsner was named president of the corporation; LeJeune and Caldwell, vice-presidents; Tyrone, secretary; and Burns, treasurer. The next day, acts of sale transferred ownership of the Physicians and Surgeons Building, purchased for $80,000; the Martin property, $12,000; and the Rice property, $9,000, to the corporation. For an outlay of $101,000, borrowed from the Hibernia Bank, the professors were getting ready to receive patients.

The architectural firm of Goldstein, Parham, and Labouisse was engaged to draw up plans for renovation of the property, and Gervais Favrot, contractor, was hired to do the work. Junius Underwood, business manager, the first lay employee of the clinic, began negotiations with tenants to clear the way for the alterations and eventual occupancy. He had been sent to observe operations at existing clinics in preparation for organizing the activities of the Ochsner group.

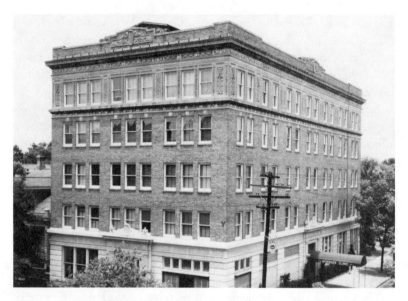

The clinic building at Aline and Prytania

Renovation was still in progress when Burns and his associate urologist, Willoughby E. Kittredge, moved in on October 1. Burns and other partners continued to see their patients as private practitioners pending the official opening of the clinic. Two months later the United States entered World War II when the Japanese attacked Pearl Harbor, but the painters, carpenters, and plasterers continued to work right through the official opening on January 2, 1942. A smiling Enid Cary, the receptionist, kept her equanimity amid the dust and din, directing the pioneer patients to their doctors' offices. Watching Cary warmly greet every visitor to the reception area during the clinic's early days, Frank Lahey told Ochsner, "Al, she's the making of the clinic."

The regional appeal of the clinic was evident from the start. First came Mrs. George Willings of Pensacola, Florida, patient number 000 001 on a list that by August, 1984, had grown to 761,606 names. Le-Jeune, who had treated her previously, diagnosed her ear problem as otitis media and marked on her admission card that there would be no charge for the visit, no doubt a recognition of the fact that she was a trailblazer. Patient number 000 002, the first to be referred by an out-side practitioner, was Anna Meeks of Hattiesburg, Mississippi. She was sent to LeJeune by Dr. Earl Green of Hattiesburg for treatment of a tumor in the nose. The first New Orleanian, registered as patient number 000 003, was sixteen-year-old William M. Barnett, who developed a thyroid problem while at home on Christmas vacation from Exeter Academy. His mother took him to the clinic to see Samuel B. Nadler, an internist and the Barnett family physician. Thus, Barnett was the first patient to be assigned to one of the nonfounder doctors on the starting staff.

Nineteen physicians were associated with the clinic when it opened. General surgeons were Ochsner, DeBakey, Matas (consultant), Mims Gage, Owens (consultant in plastic surgery), and Echols (consultant in neurosurgery). Findley led the internal medicine section, comprising Nadler, Musser (consultant), and Julius Wilson (consultant in diseases of the chest). Edgar H. Little was the staff radiologist. Guy Caldwell and Harry D. Morris covered bone and joint surgery. The obstetrics and gynecology department comprised Tyrone and John C. Weed. Burns and Kittredge made up the urology department, and LeJeune and Philip J. Bayon covered ear, nose, and throat.

Perhaps the consultant most envied by other New Orleans physicians and most eagerly enlisted by the Ochsner Clinic founders was Rudolph Matas. His reputation towered over that of every other New Orleans medical man in the closing years of the nineteenth century and the first decades of the twentieth. In the 1930s and 1940s his presence was a reminder of a bygone period when New Orleans physicians fought yellow fever, cholera, typhus, tuberculosis, bubonic plague—and often each other. His disciples, former students who had learned surgical techniques in his Tulane classes and Charity Hospital demon-strations, held him in awe.

Matas' fame rested largely on his daring thoracic and vascular surgery and his experimentation with spinal anesthesia and blood trans-fusions, but in New Orleans he was also known as an old-time physician whose province was the human skin and the contents thereof. People remembered that his efforts to bring about mosquito control in New Orleans had been the most important single factor in the con-

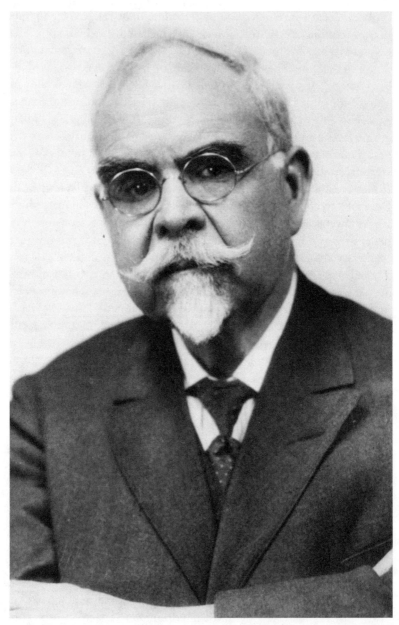

Rudolph Matas

quest of yellow fever. In the years before age and blindness ended his active career, he was a familiar figure, instantly recognizable by his white goatee as he was driven about the streets in his big sedan.

Matas had entered the New Orleans scene before 1880 as a brilliant medical student at the University of Louisiana, the school that would soon become Tulane University. He found himself in an atmosphere charged with antagonisms between French-speaking and English-speaking physicians. The differences dated back to the beginning of the century when the Louisiana Purchase in 1803 was followed by an influx of American frontiersmen looking for an opportunity to get rich quickly in a busy international port. The resident Creoles resented the intruders, and a no-man's land took shape along Canal Street between the French Quarter and the American settlement. From the American states also came physicians and surgeons attracted by the prospects of lucrative practice in a fever-ridden, subtropical city with a polyglot, disease-prone population. They competed with the Creole practitioners, some of whom had been sent by their families to study in Paris, then the medical capital of the world. A degree from Paris was so prestigious that lucky doctors who trained there signed their names with the addendum M.D.P.—Medical Doctor Paris. Resentments between Creole and American doctors went beyond language. The French school approached disease with finesse, giving minimal doses of medicine and depending on tender nursing care to help the patient's body throw off the disease. On the other hand, most of the Americans practiced heroic medicine, bleeding their patients and giving them wracking doses of calomel and quinine. Sometimes the sick person would survive.

By the time Matas launched his long and distinguished career, New Orleans was well established as a center where a patient could get up-to-date treatment. The largest city in the South attracted ambitious physicians and surgeons who would keep up with medical progress. No other town within a five-hundred-mile radius had so many practitioners with such a variety of skills. The Creole doctors introduced European therapies, and the Tulane University School of Medicine, succeeding the University of Louisiana, was entering a long period of ascendancy that led to preeminence in the South and national respect.

In fact, in 1940 Tulane was the principal reason that New Orleans kept a place on the medical map. The Louisiana State University School of Medicine, which received its first class in October, 1931, had only begun to send out the graduates who now have a lion's share of the practice in the cities and towns all over the state. Men with Tulane backgrounds—such as Urban Mayes, surgeon, and Edgar Hull, internist—filled out the LSU faculty. Tulane had its pick of local practitioners eagerly awaiting appointment to its part-time teaching staff as clinical professors or instructors. A Tulane faculty roster amounted to an honor roll of local private doctors. The students who were exposed to these men in classrooms and on hospital rounds remembered them when they encountered problems in their practices. Most of the patients who came to New Orleans for diagnosis or treatment by specialists were those who were referred to doctors on the Tulane faculty.

Normal town and gown rivalry was particularly bad in New Orleans mainly because too many physicians and surgeons tried to make careers in the city where they were trained. Not only did two medical schools produce new M.D.'s every year, but Charity Hospital and, to a somewhat lesser extent, Touro Infirmary also turned out large classes of interns and residents. Charity, with its many thousands of patients and wealth of clinical material, could take its pick of graduates from medical schools all over the country. Young doctors made professional contacts during their student and house staff years, and many elected to break into practice locally. With so many practitioners competing for patients, it was to be expected that those without faculty appointments resented the advantage of professional exposure and public prestige enjoyed by the teachers.

Making a living was difficult for doctors. The Great Depression had not yet given way to the buildup for World War II. Fees were low to begin with, and collections uncertain in pre–Blue Cross, pre-Medicare times. Merrill O. Hines recalled his practice in Tylertown, Mississippi, where he would actually receive only one-third of the amount he billed for his services. New Orleans doctors could claim results scarcely, if at all, better, and the difficulty of making collections added fuel to the jealousy of successful competitors.

Solo practice was the norm. When a young man finished his training, he would hang out his shingle and set out on his own to win patients. Prohibited from advertising, he had little choice but to wait for referrals from established colleagues while making himself readily available to his circle of friends and acquaintances. If he had a pleasant bedside manner and impressed early patients with his results and his willingness to make house calls, his reputation would be spread by word of mouth and he would be kept busy. Some new doctors would be invited to become junior associates of established physicians. They would know lean times, too, but after an apprenticeship could become full partners. It was not unusual in New Orleans for two or three physicians to operate together out of one office, usually practicing the same specialty. This kind of arrangement was not viewed as an economic threat to the rest of the medical community, but local doctors were dismayed at New Orleanians who went off to the Mayo Clinic when they were ill. The establishment of the brothers Mayo was highly esteemed among the general population and was believed to offer a level of expertise far beyond that of the ordinary physician. The public was less aware of other such institutions—the Lahey Clinic, the Henry Ford Hospital, the Cleveland Clinic, and the faculty groups at Johns Hopkins University and Duke University—but doctors knew them well and feared their impact. The logic of the team approach to diagnosis and treatment was indisputable, but the economic implications for lone practitioners were not encouraging. Some opponents even tried to have the American Medical Association denounce the plan as unethical or ban it as a form of fee splitting.

The only multispecialty group in New Orleans in 1940, the Nix Clinic on Carrollton Avenue, headed by James T. Nix, was small and did not seriously challenge traditional practice. Nevertheless, it was unpopular in medical circles. An editorial in the New Orleans *Item*, December, 1940, gave an illustration of this disapproval: "A certain learned medical organization before which the clinic wanted to exhibit some of its work and results refused to permit the exhibit as that of 'the Nix Clinic,' but found it acceptable if presented in the name of 'J. T. Nix and Associates.' There was some pernicious magic about that naughty word 'clinic' that had to be exorcised." Yet, the *Item* proclaimed, "Clinics are no longer a novelty. Some are famous."

And despite the antagonism of many solo practitioners, the Ochsner founders chose perhaps the most propitious moment of the century for starting a group practice in New Orleans. They became established just in time to take full advantage of a revolution in medical science and economics that favored the clinic approach. Within the few years just before and after the clinic's founding, the discovery of sulfa drugs, penicillin, and the whole spectrum of antibiotics gave doctors the ability to effectively treat pneumonia and other frequently fatal illnesses. For the first time, doctors could do more than simply ameliorate a patient's suffering while waiting for him to either recover or die. It had become possible to actually cure disease. The emphasis in medicine shifted toward understanding and curing such baffling ailments as cancer, arthritis, and heart disease. Effective treatment of such complex diseases required advanced training in sophisticated techniques, however. Specialization became increasingly important, and the clinic provided the patient with access to the specialists.

By the time the Ochsner clinic was opened, a new era in medical economics was also dawning. The day had not yet arrived when almost every patient was covered by health insurance or by a government program for paying his doctor's and hospital bills, but it was on the way. In the early 1930s Flint-Goodridge Hospital offered New Orleans' first hospital insurance, charging a premium of $3.65 a year. Touro Infirmary followed with a similar plan, and in 1934 Hotel Dieu, Mercy, Southern Baptist, and Touro chartered the Hospital Service Association, which in 1938 became Blue Cross. Health insurance began to have nearly universal acceptance after World War II, when it became a fringe benefit in collective labor bargaining. Medicare and Medicaid in the 1960s added coverage for millions of citizens, enabling those who formerly could not afford it to seek physicians' services and enter hospitals. In 1982 only one-tenth of the patients in the Ochsner hospital lacked health insurance that protected them against at least some of the cost of their care. If collections still had to be made hit-or-miss from patients with no insurance, the Ochsner Clinic and hospital could not have grown to their present size.

Along with the development of health programs that gave most Americans ready access to physicians came an explosion in medical research. Money from foundations and the government poured into the laboratories, from which arose discoveries that would lengthen life, but only at a price. New equipment and new therapies were as expensive as they were complex, and often they were beyond the re-

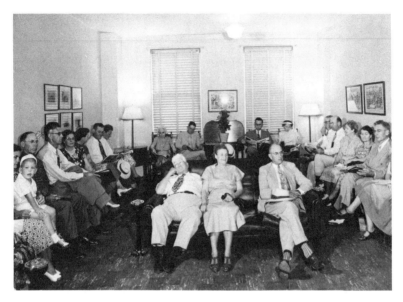

The waiting room in the first clinic building

sources of the individual physician. Some new radiological systems, for example, may cost as much as $3 million. Only the hospitals and the larger clinics can afford such investments in equipment.

Moreover, the burgeoning medical research was developing sensitive new tests that would reveal disease even before symptoms appeared. The way was cleared for the practice of preventive medicine, and most Americans could afford to take advantage of its benefits. For the first time, the healthy joined the sick in visits to doctors' offices. The annual physical checkup became a ritual for more and more Americans, and the Ochsner clinic would share this new patient load.

Ironically, the outbreak of World War II three weeks before the clinic doors swung open also provided a headstart. About two hundred New Orleans doctors—more than 25 percent—were called into the armed services, and there was an oversupply of patients for those who stayed home. But the founders of the Ochsner Clinic had all reached middle age, and the army was looking for young men.

The clinic, off to an exhilarating start, was an instant success. By the time it was two years old the busy partners had gained enough confidence in the future to venture beyond the treatment of patients and turn some of their energies to medical research, the training of young doctors, and the care of charity cases. They contributed their assets to the organization of the Alton Ochsner Medical Foundation, through which these activities were conducted. In five years the demands of patients for the services of the clinic surgeons and physicians had overwhelmed the capacity of existing private hospital facilities in New Orleans. The pressure for beds necessitated the opening of the Ochsner group's own facility, the Foundation Hospital. Then, the rapid growth of the clinic patient load coincided with the end of the war, and the partners were able to increase the medical staff rapidly by recruiting doctors who were returning from military service.

CHAPTER THREE

The Founders Plus One

The founders of the Ochsner Clinic risked ostracism by medical colleagues and put their own careers on the line in order to join together in a venture that had no guarantee of success. Neither before nor since, in the two and a half centuries that the healing arts have been practiced in New Orleans, is it likely that a group with comparable qualification could have been assembled.

All five were well established, entering middle age, with enviable professional reputations that were reflected in their prominence on the Tulane faculty. Their most productive years lay ahead, when full national and international recognition would enhance not only an individual name but also the standing of the Ochsner Clinic itself. Four of the professors brought to the association connections to some of the brightest stars in the history of New Orleans medicine. They were protégés or successors of Rudolph Matas, C. Jeff Miller, Joseph Hume, and Robert Clyde Lynch, who dominated an earlier scene. It was a noble heritage.

Alton Ochsner

If Alton Ochsner had been a soldier, he would have emerged from the wars with at least four stars on his shoulder; if an industrialist, as the president of General Motors; if a politician, as secretary of state. A winner touched by the wand of greatness, he was audacious, opportunistic, secure in his belief in what he called Presbyterian luck. His

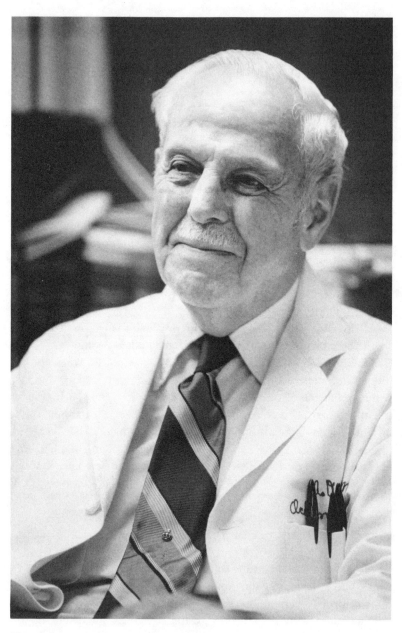

Alton Ochsner

training provided him with the skills to explore surgical frontiers. His knowledge of anatomy, physiology, pharmacology; his awareness of advances in medical science made him a memorable teacher to the many hundreds of students and young doctors who sat in his classes at Tulane or attended his demonstrations at Charity Hospital. He was born with star quality, the warm personal presence and aura of excitement that captivated public and patients and inspired trust. Yet had he not also possessed tact and respect for others' views, it is doubtful that four successful, highly individualistic associates would have subordinated their own ambitions and accepted relative anonymity in the building of institutions that bear his name.

Born at Kimball, South Dakota, on May 4, 1896, Ochsner was graduated from the University of South Dakota in 1918 and from the Washington University School of Medicine at St. Louis in 1920. A cousin, A. J. Ochsner of Chicago, the first of the name to win a wide reputation in surgery, directed his preparation. He had Alton train in internal medicine before taking him on as his surgical resident in Chicago. And he arranged for the young doctor to spend two years of surgical residency at hospitals in Switzerland and Germany.

A year of surgical practice at Chicago convinced Ochsner that he wanted to be a teacher. He was on the faculty at the University of Wisconsin when Tulane offered him the chairmanship of its surgery department. It was a controversial appointment. When Ochsner arrived in New Orleans in 1927 to take up his post he was barely past thirty. The young outsider seemed an unlikely prospect to succeed the idolized Rudolph Matas. Other more experienced surgeons, each with his own following, had hoped to pick up Matas' scalpel, and Ochsner found unfriendly rivals within his own department. The experience taught him to value his associates' loyalty above all other attributes.

As the chief Tulane surgeon at Charity Hospital, Ochsner was presented with hundreds of opportunities to prove his proficiency in the operating room. Thoracic surgery was in its infancy, and he became a pioneer in the field that interested him most. He performed, for example, the first operation in the South to remove a lung lobe. Although he was especially attracted to thoracic surgery, Ochsner also tackled many other kinds of difficult procedures, even brain surgery. In the highly visible Charity Hospital milieu, Ochsner made a new generation of medical men forget about Rudolph Matas. At the same time he was involved in research and writing that attracted further attention. By 1940, when the idea of a clinic began to take form, Ochsner had indeed become the indispensable element.

Once the clinic was opened, the Ochsner name attracted patients. Movie stars, presidents, sports champions sought him out, lending further luster to his reputation and making him a celebrity in his own right. Possibly no other man was ever honored with election to the presidencies of so many national and international medical societies. In Latin America he became a legend, and thousands of Hispanics flocked to the Ochsner institutions for treatment. In New Orleans he won the ultimate civic acclaim, ruling as Rex, king of Mardi Gras. For fourteen years after 1967, when clinic rules barred him from the operating room because of age, he continued to see patients in his office. Millions of Americans knew him as the chief foe of cigarettes, the prophet who warned that smoking causes cancer.

Ochsner was interested in the broad view and left the details of clinic administration to others. He presented his ideas but yielded gracefully to the opinions of the other founders. It was usually Ochsner who mediated when the other partners disagreed, and his diplomacy was one of the reasons the original partnership always emerged from a meeting with a unanimous vote, even when the discussion behind closed doors had been heated.

Guy Alvin Caldwell

During World War I, new orthopedic surgical techniques that enabled crippled children to throw away their buckles, braces, and belts and walk without aid began being developed. One of the pioneers of these techniques was Guy Alvin Caldwell, the surgeon who in 1922 performed the first operation at the first of the Shriners' children's hospitals to open in the United States, in Shreveport, Louisiana. As a child, Caldwell had lost the little finger of his left hand in a mill accident at Corinth, Mississippi, but the handicap did not lessen his skill as a surgeon.

But Caldwell was born with a head for business management, and

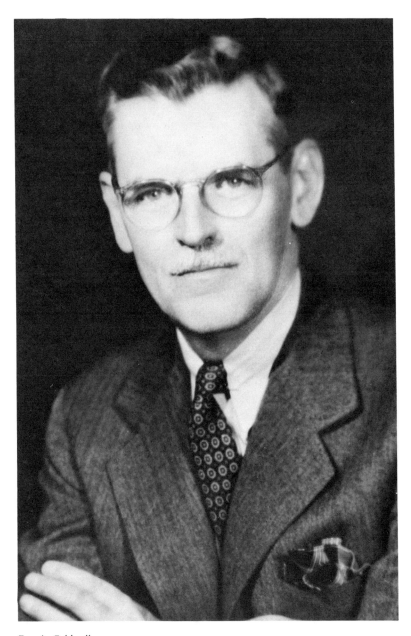

Guy A. Caldwell

throughout his career the talent sidetracked him from his purely surgical duties. In France in World War I, as adjutant of his medical unit, he had to serve as manager of an army hospital. And in Atlanta, where he returned to civilian practice, he became assistant administrator of the Henry Grady Hospital as well as instructor in fractures at Emory University. Once the Ochsner Clinic was launched, Caldwell found more and more administrative duties thrust upon him by the other partners. He had vision, along with financial acumen, and he emerged as the architect of the structure of the Ochsner Institutions. He was also, in the words of Curtis Tyrone, "the glue that held us together."

Born in Alcorn County, Mississippi, on January 24, 1891, Caldwell was graduated from the University of Mississippi, and in 1914 obtained his doctor of medicine degree from the Columbia University College of Physicians and Surgeons. He was named chief of surgery for the Shriner's Crippled Children's Hospital at Shreveport in 1922, and he also began the private practice of orthopedics in that city. The idea of group practice already intrigued him, and he attempted unsuccessfully to persuade other Shreveport doctors to join him in establishing a clinic.

On a visit to Shreveport to attend a meeting, Alton Ochsner was invited to make hospital rounds with Caldwell. Ochsner was impressed with what he saw, and the two men developed a close friendship. In 1938 Ochsner brought Caldwell to New Orleans as professor of orthopedics at Tulane. When talk of organizing a clinic made up of Tulane faculty members gained momentum in 1940, Caldwell was one of the most enthusiastic advocates.

For years he ran the orthopedic department of the clinic and performed surgery while also busying himself with fiscal affairs, staff activities, and negotiations that resulted in the present Ochsner plant. He was elected president of the American Academy of Orthopedic Surgeons and of the American Board of Orthopedic Surgery. In 1957 he gave up his practice, except for occasional consultations, to become full-time medical director.

A tall, erect man with the courtly manners of a southern planter, Caldwell exerted telling influence in partnership councils because he was the best informed of the founders and presented his views with both force and tact. He sometimes clashed with Edgar Burns, who had his own ideas about the way the clinic should be run. They might not speak to each other for a while, but eventually ruffled feelings would be mollified. Somehow the five different personalities were always able to work out their disputes without lasting scars.

Subordinates found Caldwell formal and demanding, but they knew, too, that he advocated good pay and working conditions for them, and they respected him. Accustomed to command, for three years after he stepped down as medical director, Caldwell retained a desk in the office of his successor, Merrill O. Hines, whom he did not hesitate to second-guess. It was an uncomfortable situation for Hines. But years later, when he was nearing his ninetieth birthday, Caldwell came to the hospital in his wheelchair to apologize. He broke into tears as he told Hines how sorry he was that he had given the younger man such a hard time. Hines, embracing his former boss, assured him that he had only respect and affection for the man he had always called Professor.

Edgar Burns

The elevators at the first clinic building at Prytania and Aline were balky, and often operators had difficulty stopping them at floor level. One morning Sidney Broussard, a porter, noted that a car awaiting passengers on the first floor was two or three inches too high. At the same time he spotted Edgar Burns entering from the parking lot.

"Here comes Dr. Burns," Broussard warned the operator. "You'd better get this elevator even."

"He can look down like everybody else," the woman responded.

"He ain't never yet," said Broussard.

Edgar Burns marched through the halls with back straight and head high, an unbending, authoritarian figure regarded with some apprehension by employees and younger staff members. Yet they lined up outside his office door to bring up their working problems. They might not always like his decisions, but here was one power who said yes or no immediately.

Once, a staff internist became exasperated with a patient who continually interrupted him.

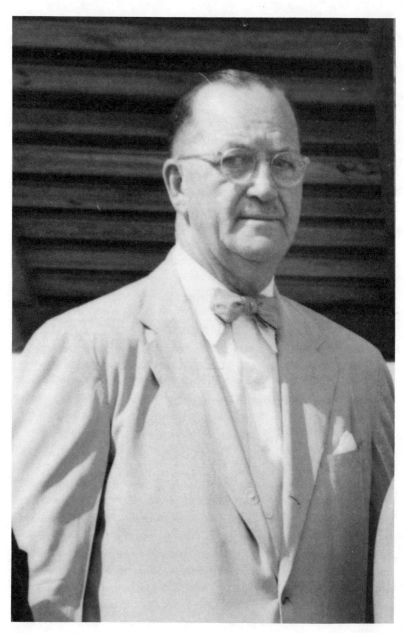

Edgar Burns

"If you'll shut your damn mouth, I'll tell you what to do," the doctor snapped.

The patient complained to Burns, who summoned the internist and summarily fired him.

On another occasion a resident in urology made a last-minute change in an operating-room schedule.

"Don't you ever make up your mind?" asked one of the anesthesiology residents.

Burns heard of the incident and fired the impatient resident.

Edgar Burns became involved in the day-by-day direction of the clinic almost by default. Ochsner, LeJeune, and Tyrone had little interest in the routine, and Caldwell was busy with planning.

The doctors and nurses who knew Burns in the years when he was one of America's most eminent urologists would have been surprised by a scene in the office of Joseph Hume during Burns's early period in New Orleans. Born at Maud, Alabama, on August 15, 1895, Burns was graduated from the University of Mississippi and obtained his doctor of medicine degree at Northwestern University in 1922. He trained and taught at the University of Tennessee before coming to New Orleans in 1928 as an assistant to Hume, one of the faculty stalwarts at the Tulane medical school and widely respected as the pioneer urologist in the city. Despite two years in the army in World War I and his rapidly developing operating room proficiency, Burns was shy. He walked with a slight stoop, perhaps to disguise how tall he was, and he was known as "good old Ed" among the young physicians with whom he gossiped over coffee after hospital rounds. He was about to leave Hume's office one day to deliver his first medical paper when Hume had a word of advice: "Stand up straight, Edgar, and speak right out." When Hume died in 1936, a change came over Burns. He took on the dignified air expected of a practitioner who had attained senior stature. But he never lost his warmth with his patients, who trusted him and kept his waiting room crowded.

Burns and Eugene Vickery carried on Hume's practice in his office in the American Bank Building until Burns made up his mind to join the group that formed the Ochsner Clinic. Each of the founders was entitled to bring in an associate as a staff member, and Burns invited Willoughby E. Kittredge to join him. "I don't know whether the clinic is going to work out," he told Kittredge. "If it blows up, you and I will go back downtown together."

Burns had his office furniture and records brought in on October 1, 1941. It was a Saturday, and Tulane was playing a football game that afternoon, but October 1 is the traditional moving day in New Orleans and Burns's lease on the American Bank office had expired. Burns and Kittredge saw patients despite the confusion of the renovation of the Physicians and Surgeons Building.

Burns's original partnership with Eugene Vickery had not been dissolved entirely amicably. There was a dispute over the patient records Burns had taken with him from Hume's office. One night, when he emerged from Touro Infirmary after making his rounds, Vickery saw a light in Burns's new office across the street. He decided to confront his former partner. Angry words soon degenerated to a fist fight, and Burns wound up with a black eye.

In bringing Burns into the clinic, the other founders not only established a link with the Hume tradition, they also gained an associate who would add prestige to the group on his own account. Edgar Burns became president of the American Board of Urology, of the Clinical Society of Gastrourinary Surgeons, and of the American Urological Association. He won the Ramon Guiteras Award of the American Urological Association and the Keyes Gold Medal of the American Association of Gastrourinary Surgeons. His death on August 27, 1973, was the first break in the ranks of the founders.

Francis E. LeJeune

Francis Ernest LeJeune used to lament, half-jokingly: "Until I went into the clinic I didn't have an enemy. Now I'm an SOB." But this hardworking, fun-loving Cajun more often shrugged off the occasional snubs he received from fellow physicians. In the heady days when the Ochsner Clinic began attracting national attention, LeJeune was one of its most visible assets. One of the giants of ear, nose, and throat medicine, he became the second doctor in history to win all three major ENT prizes—the Casselberry, Newcomb, and deRoaldes awards—and he served as president of the Triological Society, the American Laryn-

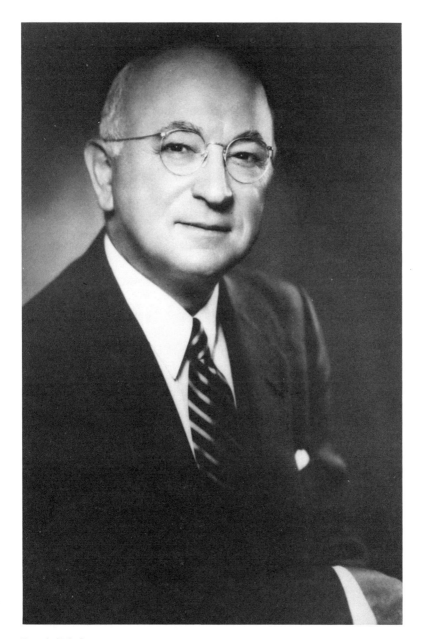

Francis E. LeJeune

gological Assocition, the American Academy of Ophthalmology and Otolaryngology, and the American Broncho-Esophagological Association. He pioneered the use of color motion pictures in laryngology and helped perfect suspension laryngoscopic techniques. He also brought a steady flow of patients to the newly opened offices at Aline and Prytania streets, for he was in the mainstream of New Orleans health activities.

LeJeune completed his residency at the Eye, Ear, Nose, and Throat Hospital in New Orleans, which was founded by A. W. deRoaldes, for whom the award he later won was named. He had an offer to join a practitioner at Mobile, and his fiancée, Anna Lynne Dodds, was agreeable to living in the Alabama city. He had made up his mind to move there when Robert Clyde Lynch, the most respected otolaryngologist in the South, invited him to become a partner. Afterward, all paths led upward. He began teaching part-time at Tulane, and in 1931 he inherited most of Lynch's patients when the latter was killed in an automobile accident.

Few doctors have lived a fuller life than LeJeune did before his death on October 13, 1977, at eighty-three. His wife and close friends called him Bobilo, but his colleagues dubbed him Duke de Thibodaux in acknowledgment of the small Louisiana town where he was born on August 26, 1894. LeJeune's father was a sugar engineer, whose work took the family to Mexico for a year and Puerto Rico for three years. During this time LeJeune added Spanish to the French and English he had already learned to speak in his bilingual Acadian household.

After a stint as an army private during World War I, LeJeune entered Tulane University as an engineering student, but after three years he switched to medicine because, he said, he found the mathematics unfathomable. A perfectionist, he was fond of saying, "If a thing is worth doing, it is worth doing right. If it is not worth doing right, don't waste time on it." It was a philosophy that helped set the pattern of procedure in Ochsner operating rooms. His son, Francis, Jr., joined his father's department in 1959, and the elder LeJeune was on edge when the young man's first solo surgery was scheduled. "Now we'll know," he told Anna LeJeune. When the procedure went well, he was walking on air. Long after he had to retire from active surgery at the age of seventy, LeJeune continued to spend hours watching others operate, offering advice when asked. Up until his death, he delighted in extending his right arm to demonstrate how steady his hand still was.

Not long after Alton Ochsner settled in New Orleans, he was attending a medical meeting in El Paso, Texas, when he had a telephone call from Isabel Ochsner, who told him their older sons, Alton, Jr., and John, had undergone mastoid operations performed by LeJeune. It took Ochsner thirty-six anxious hours to get home by train. Isabel met him at the station and drove him to Touro Infirmary, where he encountered LeJeune for the first time. "As soon as I met him, I relaxed," Ochsner related years later. "I knew our boys were in good hands."

The LeJeunes frequently saw Alton and Isabel Ochsner socially, and sometimes the Ochsners joined them on fishing trips on LeJeune's boat. Long afterward, Anna LeJeune recalled that Ochsner had told her husband before the clinic was founded, "If you don't come in, I'll drop the matter."

LeJeune shared equally with the other founders in income from the clinic, but he was perhaps the most successful in outside investments. He was a schoolmate of the New Orleans banker and financier, Louis Roussel. When Roussel, then a streetcar conductor, was first dabbling in oil leases, he borrowed fifty dollars from LeJeune to close a deal. It was the first of several loans from LeJeune that helped Roussel get started. Later he made the surgeon a director in some of his businesses.

LeJeune won enough professional acclaim to slake the thirst for fame of the most ambitious medical men, yet he was willing to take a place largely obscured from the public eye by the shadow of Alton Ochsner. Like the other founders, he had a vision of an institution greater than the combined genius of the men who created it. He had no regrets over the career he chose.

Curtis Tyrone

Curtis Hartman Tyrone was the workhorse of the founder group. He also became the maverick, sometimes threatening to pull out of the clinic and resume solo practice because he was seeing patients day and night while the other partners were spending part of their time teaching or going off to medical meetings. Tyrone himself usually avoided

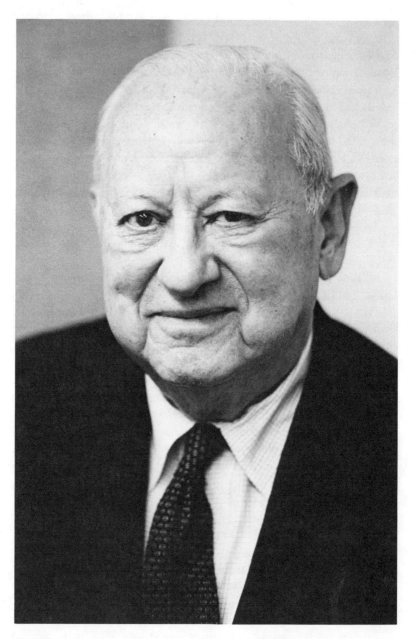

Curtis Tyrone

professional gatherings. "I'm no orator," he expalined. He was aware of the fact that as a result, his national recognition among his peers was less than that enjoyed by the other clinic founders, and he was sensitive about it. When Guy Caldwell wrote the first history of the clinic, he planned to include a curriculum vita of each of the founders. Tyrone put a stop to the idea, threatening a lawsuit if necessary, because he felt his short list of outside affiliations and activities would reflect unfairly upon him. Yet among New Orleanians in need of an obstetrician or gynecologist, his reputation was second to none.

Born at Prentiss, Mississippi, on April 18, 1898, Tyrone as a boy chopped cotton to help support his family. At Mississippi College his ambition was to become a professor of history, but instead he entered the Tulane medical school, from which he was graduated in 1923. He was completing his internship at Touro Infirmary when, on June 15, 1925, came "the luckiest day of my life."

"There I was, with no money and without the slightest idea of where I would be able to practice," he recalled. "That afternoon, as we were making the hospital rounds, Dr. [Charles] Jefferson Miller asked, 'Are you busy?' I told him no and he asked me to walk to his automobile with him. When we got there he inquired, 'What are you going to do on July 1?' My internship was ending, and I admitted I had no prospects. Then he said, 'Can you come into my office and work with me?' I said yes without even asking him if I'd earn as much as 15 cents a month."

As matters turned out, it was a fortunate day for the future Ochsner Clinic as well as for Tyrone. "If you drew a line from Galveston, Texas, to Jacksonville, Florida, Dr. Miller was *the* gynecologist," Tyrone remarked. Miller was destined to become president of the American Gynecological Society in 1928 and the American College of Surgeons in 1931. His professional abilities won him the busiest ob-gyn practice in New Orleans, and his personality made him a leader in medical circles. Because of his association with Miller, the younger Tyrone brought into the clinic not only an officeful of well-to-do leaders of society but also prestige that was valuable in the early days.

But affiliation with Miller proved to be no quick road to riches. "The first years were hell financially," Tyrone remembered. He did not see patients as an assistant to the busy gynecologist, but instead took care of the overflow, covered for Miller when the latter was away, and began building up a practice of his own. Miller saw the potential in the ambitious, energetic young doctor with his deftness and finesse in the operating room and an affable personality for charming women of all ages, from young wives with their first pregnancies to dowagers with late-life gynecological problems. Later, surgeons who worked with him would describe a Tyrone operation as a symphony, an artistic as well as an effective performance.

In the early 1930s Miller's younger brother, Hilliard E. Miller, shared an office with Jeff and Tyrone. Friction developed between the brothers, and Hilliard Miller decided to pull out of the affiliation. He asked Tyrone to join him. Jeff Miller, who never called his protégé by his first name, told the young doctor: "Tyrone, you're twenty-one years old, and you can make up your own mind. But if you leave me, it will be like having a knife stuck in my heart." Tyrone was touched.

"Dr. Jeff," he replied, "if you'll let me stay, I'll never leave you." He later described the encounter as a "very, very beautiful experience." When Jeff Miller died on March 21, 1936, Tyrone inherited most of his patients and succeeded him as the city's leading gynecologist. He began teaching gynecology on a part-time basis at Tulane University in 1925 and continued until 1964.

Preoccupied with his practice, Tyrone did not hear the rumblings about the move among other members of the Tulane medical faculty to organize a clinic until he was approached in early 1940 by his friend, Edgar Burns. "Al Ochsner and Guy Caldwell have asked me to join in a group," Burns informed Tyrone. "I told them I would consider it, but there is one condition. I won't come in unless you also invite Curtis Tyrone." The others were agreeable to the thought of adding Tyrone's lucrative uptown practice to the clinic's potential clientele. For his part, Tyrone cast his lot with the group because Burns wanted him in.

Tyrone always said he paid a higher price than any of the others for coming into a group that stirred up so much animosity. "I had more friends in the medical profession here than the others did. Some of them never spoke to me again." Willoughby E. Kittredge was playing poker with a table of doctors at Tyrone's home, at Prytania and Valence streets, on the night the bag with the thirty pieces of silver was delivered to each founder. "Dr. Tyrone answered the doorbell," Kittredge related. "When he came back he was red in the face, but he never said a word."

As the youngest of the founders, Tyrone was the most likely to be drafted into the armed services in 1943 when a drive for doctors was being made. Army representatives met with officers of the Orleans Parish Medical Society in January to determine how many physicians and surgeons could be recruited without crippling the city's medical services. The word spread that every doctor under forty-five would have to go. Tyrone would be forty-five on April 18. He went to see C. Grenes Cole, chairman of a medical society committee that was working with the armed services. The identities of two other members of the committee were kept secret. Cole told Tyrone, "You're doing a great job. You go back to work. We're actually not taking anybody over thirty-eight now." After the war, one of the anonymous committee members confided, "You'd be surprised at the telegrams and calls we received from doctors who wanted to get you into the service." Tyrone concluded that the unfriendly doctors "figured that was the only way they could break up the Ochsner Clinic."

The demand for medical services was so pressing in 1943 that during the entire year Tyrone did not leave the East Bank city limits of New Orleans, did not even cross the river to Algiers. He continued his habits of hard work until his retirement in 1968. Once, he submitted a bill to the clinic for $7.50 for half-soling shoes he said he wore out while attending patients. On November 19, 1951, he sent a handwritten note to the administrative committee: "At the end of the month I will have completed eleven months of work here with only 3 days off— one Tuesday and two Saturdays. I have had no vacation and no trips and I am requesting the Ochsner Clinic to defray my expenses to the coming meeting of the Southern Surgical Association." Despite an occasional temper flare-up when he complained that he and Burns were carrying most of the work load, Tyrone was glad that he went into the clinic.

A minor mystery surrounded Tyrone after the present campus was opened. Clinic officials noticed that his radiation badge continued to record heavy doses even though Tyrone had not been near the X-ray rooms or anywhere else where he might have been exposed to radiation. At last an explanation was uncovered. In his desk was found a missing vial of radium. How it got there, nobody knew. Like the other founders, Curtis Tyrone lived a long life, dying in 1982 in his eighty-third year.

The Sixth Founder

Nobody had more faith in the future of the Ochsner institutions than the neurosurgeon Dean H. Echols. Shrugging off the refusal of the five originators to let him come in as a partner from the start, he moved into the clinic building as soon as it was ready and kept part-time office hours as a consultant for several months before he joined up as a senior staff member. In the year before his retirement in 1975 he became both the most controversial and one of the most loyal Ochsner doctors, a ringleader in agitation that finally caused a reorganization of the partnership and a visionary who demanded action on his ideas.

In the 1960s Echols told Merrill O. Hines, the medical director, that the institutions owed him $95,000, his out-of-pocket outlay for social entertainment over the years in furthering the Ochsner activities. He proposed that he be repaid at a rate of $12,000 a year. Hines turned him down, but the suggestion was a reminder of Echols' unique contributions as the "sixth founder."

Born at Appleton, Wisconsin, on April 28, 1904, the son of a physician, Echols was graduated from Brown University and the University of Michigan medical school. He joined the Michigan faculty and wrote the second paper ever published on the surgical repair of the ruptured spinal disc. His would have been the first such report had not his department chief held it back for months because the ideas were so revolutionary. Echols was impressed with Alton Ochsner, whom he encountered at surgical meetings, and applied for a place on the Tulane faculty. Ochsner replied that there was no provision in the Tulane budget for paying him but suggested that Echols could probably establish a busy practice in New Orleans, for neurosurgery was still almost unknown in the South. Echols moved in 1937 and while serving without pay at Tulane built up his reputation as a surgeon.

Even before he became a full-time staff member, Echols began to worry about the problems of keeping the clinic thriving. From a pam-

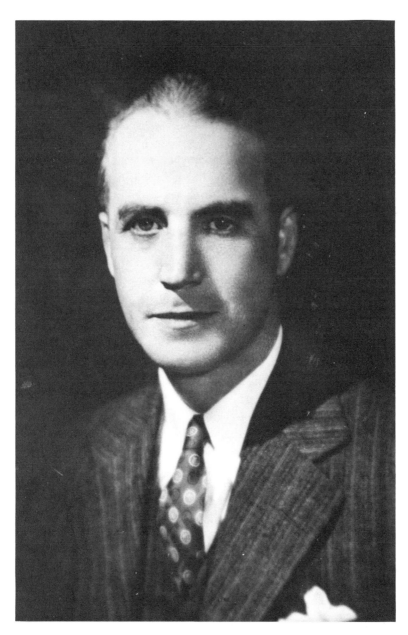

Dean Echols

phlet of the United States Public Health Service he learned that more than half of the many group practices established in this country had disappeared. The record added to his concerns, which he discussed at evening get-togethers with Junius Underwood, the clinic's business manager, who lived near Echols in the Garden District. Finally, Echols recalls, "I decided to visit the largest clinic of them all and try to learn the secret of its success." Entirely on his own, paying his own way and without consulting any of the founders, he spent a week examining the functioning of the Mayo Clinic at Rochester, Minnesota. "I became convinced," he recalled, "that if the Ochsner Clinic was to be successful, it would have to become affiliated with a non-profit medical foundation." He persuaded Underwood, and together they had a meeting, unbeknownst to the partners, with Blanc Monroe. For more than an hour, Monroe listened. Then he reminded his visitors that he was the attorney for the founders, that they expected him to look after their financial interests, and that he intended to do just that. Echols and Underwood heard no more about the matter until they learned the partners were contemplating a foundation.

On another visit to the Mayo Clinic, Echols encountered Merrill Hines, who had been sent there to study colon and rectal surgery preparatory to establishing a department at Ochsner. Hines mentioned to Echols that one of the latter's New Orleans patients had entered Mayo to undergo spinal surgery. "I'll see about that," responded Echols. He visited the man, wrote on his chart that the patient was leaving Mayo, arranged for his discharge, and admitted him to the Touro Infirmary for surgery, which Echols performed himself upon his return to New Orleans. Hines expected the chief neurosurgeon at Mayo to be upset. Instead, the doctor laughed and said: "That's Dean Echols for you. You know how he is."

When he was invited to work full-time on the staff, Echols told Guy Caldwell he wanted to be put in charge of Ochsner's program for training residents. As soon as the foundation was organized, he became education director, charged with getting the teaching activities underway. Once, in 1950 or 1951 when the patient load dropped and the clinic was in financial difficulties, Echols was one of the two or three staff members who were asked not to draw their salaries, and he lived on credit for two or three months.

When the inevitable discontent developed because staff pay was low, Echols as always was outspoken. One night the physicians and surgeons held a meeting in the clinic lobby, and each man had his say. Monroe was angered by a report of the meeting, and a day or so later the medical director, Hiram W. Kostmayer, called Echols into his office and told him he was in danger of being fired. "I don't remember taking it too seriously," Echols remarked years later. Apparently, his position had been misunderstood. He had talked about the need for higher pay, but he had also warned against action that would destroy the clinic. In any case, "there never was any talk of a strike," he related. "Too many of the staff were determined to stay, come hell or high water." Any honor roll of the men and women who made the institutions prosper would have Echols' name near the top.

CHAPTER FOUR

The Ochsner Foundation

Two years after it began operations, the Ochsner Clinic was one of the busiest medical facilities in the South. At the beginning of 1944, with the prospects of an American victory becoming brighter every day, the time had come to expand activities into areas of public service about which the Tulane professors had high hopes. There were contributions to be made in medical education, research, and charity. The founders talked about forming an association to conduct all of the Ochsner activities. But on the advice of J. Blanc Monroe, they elected to maintain the clinic for the practice of medicine and set up a nonprofit foundation to carry out all of the other functions in which they wanted to be engaged. It was an arrangement they would sometimes regret.

On January 15, 1944, before notary Watts K. Leverich, the Alton Ochsner Medical Foundation was chartered. Article II spelled out the reasons for its existence.

> The general purpose of this corporation shall be scientific, educational, literary and charitable; and to promote medical, surgical and scientific learning, skill, education and research in the broadest sense; and to aid and advance the study and investigaion of human ailments and injuries and the causes, prevention, relief and cure thereof, without distinction as to the means of the patient, his race or domicile; to provide more and better care for patients with no means and those with moderate means and to endeavor to make the care and attention to such patients equal to that given patients with the most ample means; to conduct more research, both clinical and laboratory, and in that connection to establish and operate medical libraries and museums; to provide fellowships for approved

young physicians, who have had at least one year of acceptable hospital training in order to enable them to continue their studies and research; to make available increased teaching personnel for Class A medical schools. Its further purposes shall be to purchase and acquire property and receive and administer donations of money, property or other things of value for scientific, literary, and educational purposes; to receive by purchase, gift, bequest, or in any other lawful manner, any real or personal property, to hold, use, manage, operate, lease, convey, convert, invest and dispose of by gift, sale, lease or otherwise, such property in any lawful manner for the furtherance of its general purposes, including the establishment and administration of any trust funds, the management and operation of clinics, hospitals, infirmaries and research laboratories and their accessories; the employment of and payment of reasonable compensation to physicians, surgeons, technicians, research assistants, and other employees, commensurate with their professional ability and the time and effort expended by them, the nature of the case and the skill required, the granting and financing of research fellowships and graduate certificates, and the ownership, erection and administration of physical facilities incident to the accomplishment of these purposes; and to do and perform generally and anywhere all acts and things reasonably incident to the corporation purposes and objects, including the receipt, establishment, augmentation and administration of any fund or funds which may be reasonably advantageous or convenient to the carrying out of the corporate purposes. No part of the net earnings of said corporation shall inure to the benefit of any private individual, but same shall be devoted exclusively to the advancement and promotion of its scientific, educational, charitable and literary purposes. The powers of the corporation shall be all such as are reasonably necessary to the accomplishment of these purposes and all such as may be exercised by a corporation organized under the above referred to statutes of the State of Louisiana.

If Leverich had to read the article aloud, he must have been out of breath when he finished.

Article III of the charter named the slate of officers of the foundation. Alton Ochsner was president. Duke LeJeune and Guy Caldwell were both vice-presidents. Curtis Tyrone began as treasurer, and Edgar Burns, as secretary, but at the first meeting they swapped jobs. Article III also provided for a board of trustees, five members of which were to be physicians—the founders, of course, at first. The sixth trustee was to be a "competent and experienced attorney." Without discussion, the physician members knew that J. Blanc Monroe would be the lawyer trustee.

In his office hung a framed motto: "The tendency to persevere, to persist in spite of hindrances, discouragements and impossibilities, it is this that in all things distinguishes the strong soul from the weak." The Ochsner founders soon discovered they had enlisted a strong soul as the attorney for the clinic and attorney-trustee for the foundation. In truth, they awakened to the realization that they held a tiger by the tail. More than any other man, and sometimes to the dismay of the partners, Monroe shaped the Ochsner Institutions. He wanted an institution that would merit generous public support by its high purpose and medical proficiency, and he got it. Sometimes he prevailed over the contrary opinion of all five founders.

While the clinic was being organized Caldwell remarked that "we should have an outstanding lawyer." Tyrone proposed one or two of his friends, but Caldwell believed Monroe was the best choice. The patrician New Orleanian, son of a former chief justice of the Louisiana Supreme Court, was as respected professionally in legal circles as the partners were in the medical community. He was a member of the firm of Monroe and Lemann, with offices in the Whitney Bank Building, where many of the early meetings of the Ochsner group were held. Monroe cleared his appointment with the board of administrators of Tulane University, on which he sat. A meticulous man, he made sure none of his colleagues believed a conflict of interest might exist.

"Mr. Monroe didn't know anything at first about running a clinic," Tyrone recalled. "But he soon learned." Once he did, Tyrone related, "he was dictatorial. Sometimes at a meeting, one of us would make a suggestion. 'I disagree,' Mr. Monroe said. 'If you don't do as I say, get yourself another lawyer.'" On occasion the partners would get together in advance of a meeting with Monroe and agree to confront him. But once they were face to face, the doctors often lost their resolve. Sometimes one of the partners would instruct Edgar J. Saux, then business manager, to raise a controversial issue when there was doubt about Monroe's reaction. This approach did not endear Saux to the attorney, who would go for weeks without speaking directly to him. At meetings, Monroe would aim remarks that he intended for Saux at Caldwell or somebody else. It was up to Saux to get the message.

At one time Monroe proposed that staff physicians and surgeons be hired under contracts that would prohibit them from setting up private practices in the New Orleans metropolitan area for five years if they left Ochsner. It was one Monroe proposal that the founders could not accept. They rejected the idea, and no restrictions have ever been imposed on anyone who resigned.

Largely at Monroe's insistence, the clinic and the foundation remained separate entities. When the formation of the foundation was being discussed in 1943, the attorney opined that Louisiana law forbade the practice of medicine by an association. He held to this opinion later when Caldwell and the other partners wanted to put all of the operations under one umbrella, with an arrangement for staff doctors to be paid salaries by the foundation. Monroe always blocked the change, with the result that the clinic doctors at times bore a disproportionate share of the financial burden of the foundation.

For nearly twenty years, until his death on April 20, 1960, at the age of eighty, Monroe set the course for the institutions. He devised the legal frameworks of the clinic and foundation, he took the lead in the organization of the first Ochsner hospital at Camp Plauché, and his guidance was rewarded with the development of the present campus. "He made this organization hold together," said Tyrone. The auditorium in the Ochsner Foundation Hospital is named in his honor. Upon his death, his place on the board of trustees of the foundation was taken by his son, Malcolm L. Monroe. J. Thomas Lewis, the husband of his granddaughter, has served as president and chairman of the board of the foundation.

The seventh member of the board of trustees, as provided in Article III, was to be a "competent business man experienced in handling large affairs." By this time, Blanc Monroc had excited the interest of Theodore Brent in the phenomenon that was causing such a stir among the doctors of New Orleans. Brent was just the sort of businessman envisioned in the charter.

Born at Muscatine, Iowa, on March 30, 1874, Brent left school after the seventh grade to begin working as a railroad stenographer. He came to the city in 1914 as general manager of the New Orleans Joint Traffic Bureau, beginning a thirty-nine-year-long stay in which he was one of the principal movers and shakers of his time. One of the founders of the Mississippi Shipping Company, he served as president and, later, chairman of the board. He was president of Louisiana Shipyards, and of the Hemisphere Trading Company. As a director of the Hibernia National Bank and because of his activities in the Mississippi Shipping Company, he was an associate of Rudolf S. Hecht, the banker who arranged the early financing of the clinic. Brent was also the first president of the International Trade Mart, and at one time served as chairman of the board of the Mississippi Valley Association.

Like Monroe, Brent was a hardworking trustee. He took an active part in negotiations with Tulane University and Touro Infirmary looking toward the construction of a hospital as a joint venture. Brent helped put together the arrangements that resulted in the first Ochsner hospital at Camp Plauché. In 1952, when a drive for public contributions to begin constructing the present facilities was lagging, Brent provided a spur with a $400,000 matching funds donation.

When Brent, a bachelor, died on June 8, 1953, he left the first bequest of more than a million dollars ever received by the Ochsner Foundation. His estate was appraised at $1,603,817. In his honor, the Jefferson House Hotel on the Ochsner campus was given its present name, Brent House.

Twice a year the foundation pays homage to its benefactor. At Easter, Charles Heim, the director of development, places a bouquet of calla lilies on Brent's grave in the Garden of Memories, and on All Saints' Day, a bouquet of chrysanthemums.

At the first meeting of the board of trustees, on January 17, the Ochsner Clinic, Inc., the property-holding adjunct to the clinic partnership, was dissolved. The founders donated its assets, listed as slightly less than $300,000, minus $135,000 owed to the Hibernia Bank, to the foundation. Each of the five also gave $4,300 in cash to the foundation, and collectively they donated $128,500 in notes owed to them by Ochsner Clinic, Inc. Alton Ochsner was authorized to arrange a mortgage loan of $135,000 from the Hibernia Bank to take the place of the Ochsner Clinic loan.

The founders and other clinic staff members were soon busy carrying out the charitable functions of the new foundation. Patients came from all over the Deep South and from Latin America, obviously attracted by the reputation of the Ochsner doctors. They were put into

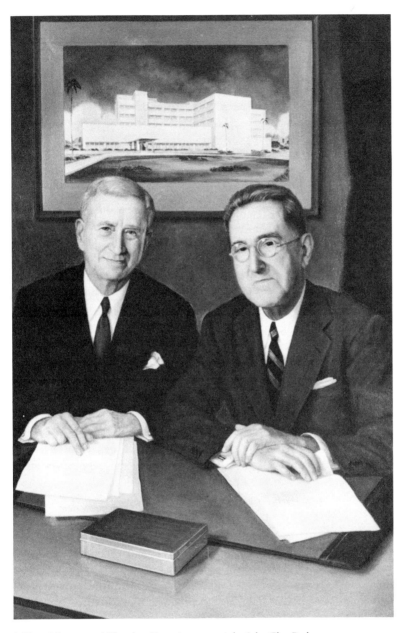

J. Blanc Monroe and Theodore Brent in a portrait by John Clay Parker beds at Touro Infirmary paid for by the foundation and given medical or surgical treatment without charge. For their part, the patients provided good opportunities for the staff to demonstrate interesting cases to the doctors in the new fellowship training program. The range of medical problems was as wide as the patients' geographical spread.

Dean H. Echols effected a surgical cure for a Yazoo City, Mississippi, woman with facial neuralgia. Willoughby E. Kittredge operated on a Donaldsonville, Louisiana, woman who had cancer of the bladder. Rawley Penick did a series of operations that benefited a ten-year-old boy with Hirschsprung's disease, a problem of the colon. The kidney of a twelve-year-old Hattiesburg, Mississippi, boy was removed, and a brain problem diagnosed for a four-year-old Springhill, Lousiana, lad. Penicillin, just coming into use, saved the life of an eighteen-year-old Jackson, Louisiana, girl with actinomycosis, a mass in the chest and neck that in those days was almost always fatal. Alton Ochsner removed the gall bladder of a fifty-one-year-old missionary from Granada, Nicaragua. A fourteen-year-old boy from Garyville, Florida, who swallowed a button that stuck in his throat underwent a gastrostomy, done by Champ Lyons, so he could be fed, and Francis E. LeJeune removed the button.

An eighteen-year-old New Orleans girl, the survivor of Siamese twins separated at birth, underwent a bilateral transplant of the ureter. A forty-four-year-old Douglas, Georgia, widow came in for treatment of ringing of the ears but refused an operation. A satisfactory convalescence was reported for a thirty-three-year-old Foxworth, Mississippi, housewife, who had a neurofibroma resected. Ochsner removed a lung lobe from a forty-five-year-old Bailey, Mississippi, log cutter with bronchiectasis. A gynecological procedure aided a Thomasville, Alabama, mother of eight. A forty-two-year-old Baton Rouge spinster had the care of three staff men. John C. Weed did a hysterectomy, Guy Caldwell removed her patella, and Paul DeCamp removed moles from her skin. Rawley Penick's exploration of the adrenals was not helpful to a twenty-five-year-old New Orleans housewife with a glandular condition, but a thirty-seven-year-old Plaquemine, Louisiana, housewife was successfully treated for endocarditis and heart failure. A cervical ganglionectomy performed by Homer D. Kirgis helped a sixty-six-year-old Loxley, Alabama, woman who had a facial nerve problem.

And Alton Ochsner used thoracoplasty to help a forty-year-old New Orleans man with pulmonary tuberculosis.

Not long after its formation, the Alton Ochsner Foundation was faced with its first major challenge. The same success that had made the foundation possible was creating a problem for the clinic. It was beginning to be strangled by a shortage of hospital beds for its patients. In New Orleans private hospitals provided barely 2,000 beds for paying customers, not as many all told as the 2,456 that Charity Hospital then maintained for those whose low incomes entitled them to treatment at state expense. Ochsner staff doctors found themselves denied the privilege of using available beds at some hospitals where they had previously been welcomed. Professional antagonisms prevailed, and clinic doctors were dropped from the courtesy staffs of several of the eleven private hospitals. As a result, Ochsner patients from out of town sometimes were told they needed surgery, then had to return home untreated because of the lack of accommodations. Some didn't come back. The growth of the clinic might have been permanently stunted had not Touro Infirmary made available a share of its 424 beds. The founders and almost all of the other clinic doctors were on the Tulane faculty. They had long enjoyed staff privileges at Touro and were not turned away in their time of need. The ties between Touro and Tulane were too close for that. Yet the Ochsner clinicians were competing for space against the rest of the Touro staff, and a confrontation was inevitable. It came later.

The bombs were still falling in Europe and the Pacific on July 8, 1944, when the trustees of the Alton Ochsner Foundation gathered, as they often did, at Blanc Monroe's home on Audubon Place to conduct the first formal meeting on the hospital dilemma. It had become clear, Lahey's advice to the contrary, that the Ochsner group would have to find a way of assuring themselves an adequate number of hospital beds by becoming involved in running a hospital. Two possibilities came under discussion. The group could either organize its own hospital, or it could join Tulane in establishing a university hospital. Nobody disputed the idea that there was a critical shortage of hospital space in New Orleans, that some three hundred additional beds were urgently needed. The trustees also knew that the foundation's programs of graduate medical education, research, and charity work could not be carried out without a hospital. Theodore Brent announced that he was prepared to contribute $100,000, and possibly more, toward a building.

Ochsner and Caldwell went to Washington to seek the advice of Basil McLean, former director of Touro Infirmary, who then was a medical corps colonel serving as a consultant. He discussed the costs of hospital construction and the means of raising funds. At another meeting on August 11, the foundation trustees explored the possibility of persuading Tulane to build a hospital at which all faculty members, including the Ochsner affiliates, could practice. The trustees were willing for the foundation to operate the hospital, if necessary, and even to absorb any operating deficits. The ideas were discussed with Hiram W. Kostmayer, acting dean of the Tulane medical school, who was destined to join the Ochsner clinic later as medical director. Negotiations proceeded far enough that on one occasion Kostmayer went to Dallas in quest of Public Works Administration financing for a university hospital, but by then the public funds were no longer available.

Efforts to work out an arrangement with either Tulane or Touro, including the proposal of an Ochsner wing at Touro, met failure in 1945. The progress of Hill-Burton legislation through Congress gave hope of financial support by the federal government for a future permanent hospital. The immediate shortage, however, was the problem. Clinic records at the time showed that 28 patients needing emergency surgery and 280 awaiting elective procedures could not be admitted to hospitals.

Then, in November, two months after the Japanese surrender, federal authorities announced offers to sell as surplus property the facilities of three temporary military hospitals. One of these, a small naval unit on the New Orleans lakefront near Bayou St. John, was unsuitable for a private facility. But the 105-acre LaGarde Hospital, on the lakefront between Canal Boulevard and the New Basin Canal, and the 71-acre station hospital for Camp Plauché, situated on the east bank of the Mississippi River in Jefferson Parish in the shadow of the Huey P. Long Bridge, offered possibilities. The thousand-bed LaGarde property, which enjoyed good transit service from the New Orleans business district, was the most desirable, and in January, 1946, the Ochsner Foundation made its bid.

At a conference in Washington with Major General Paul R. Hawley and Paul Magnuson of the Veterans Administration, Ochsner trustees asked to purchase or lease 250 beds and some of the LaGarde buildings. It was then that they discovered they had a rival bidder: the New Orleans Medical Foundation. Seventy physicians and surgeons, returning from military service, had organized the foundation for the purpose of helping veterans to reestablish their civilian practices. Of course, veterans enjoyed priority in dealing with the Veterans Administration and the War Assets Administration, but General Hawley suggested to the Ochsner representatives that the LaGarde facilities were ample to accommodate both groups if they would combine their projects.

On February 2 the Ochsner trustees formally proposed to the New Orleans Medical Foundation a plan under which five hundred LaGarde beds would be set aside as a governmental facility for the treatment of veterans, and the rest would be operated jointly by the two foundations for private patients. Charles B. Odom, who had served as chief surgeon for the armored force of General George S. Patton and who would later be elected to multiple terms as the Jefferson Parish coroner, soon emerged as the chief spokesman for the New Orleans Medical Foundation. It was Odom who notified the Ochsner Foundation trustees on February 15 that their plan had been rejected because, he argued, only about half of the members of the veterans' foundation would be able to have staff privileges under such an arrangement. Odom's group used its muscle, instead, to take over exclusive control of a section of LaGarde given over to private patients. Under the name Lakeshore Hospital, the facility was opened on June 1 with 175 beds, operating rooms, delivery rooms, and a nursery. Jilted, the Ochsner staff nevertheless sent some of its patients to Lakeshore while the trustees turned their efforts toward trying to win the remaining hospital, the second choice, Camp Plauché.

Two consultants, Basil MacLean and Lawrence J. Bradley of Rochester, New York, made a study and reported that potential earnings from Plauché would be "sufficient to cover all operating expense and also to amortize within a reasonable period the cost of conversion." They suggested that 300 of the 800 beds be put into use. The trustees began negotiations for the lease or purchase of 250 beds and equipment. This time, Ochsner called upon his friends in high places—two staff members who were on military duty in Washington, Colonel Michael E.

DeBakey of the surgeon general's office and Lieutenant Colonel Harry Brown of the Veterans Bureau. Meanwhile, Caldwell carried on talks with the Illinois Central Railroad leading to lease of the seventy-six-acre site that had been taken over by the government for the duration of the war.

In the summer of 1946 prospects for acquiring the hospital seemed so bright that the trustees appointed Major Charles Holmes, officer in charge of the army buildings and equipment, acting hospital director. Architect Collins Diboll and the contractor firm of Gervais Favrot were engaged to draw plans for converting the physical plant for civilian use. The site was obtained on a three-year lease at $7,683 a year. On October 2 a formal offer of $150,000 for buildings and equipment was announced. Then came a surprise. The newspapers reported the New Orleans Medical Foundation had bid $160,000. After thwarting the Ochsner Foundation's efforts to obtain LaGarde Hospital, Odom's organization now was moving to deny them Camp Plauché as well.

Odom claimed that the Lakeshore Hospital needed the equipment from Plauché. He also maintained that New Orleans had a surplus of hospital beds running 300 to 325 a day. Privately, however, Odom admitted to fear that if Ochsner's opened a hospital, Touro Infirmary would lose 130 patients brought in by Ochsner Clinic staff. Touro would then take patients away from Lakeshore, and the doctors in the New Orleans Medical Foundation would lose $150,000 that they had invested in Lakeshore. The big rush expected at Lakeshore had not materialized. When the civilian facility was first opened, the patient population had averaged 120 a day, but now it had dwindled to between 90 and 100. The hospital needed 100 to break even.

The New Orleans *Item* took Odom to task in an editorial entitled "Stop Obstruction at Plauché Hospital." Odom, said the newspaper, was doing the community a grave disservice by saying New Orleans did not need another hospital simply because Lakeshore was not being used to capacity. It quoted Odom as remarking, "We—who got what we asked in the way of hospital facilities—will try to block any other group from securing what they want in that respect." The *Item* commented, "This is not a pretty phrasing of the issue," and insisted, "New Orleans does need hospital facilities." The newspaper said its own survey showed that only Lakeshore Hospital was reporting no shortage

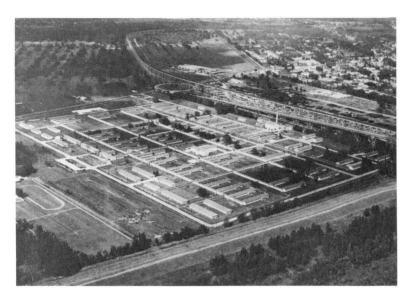

Aerial view of Splinter Village

of beds. Touro, Baptist, Hotel Dieu, Mercy, and French hospitals were all full.

Odom withdrew his offer on October 10. On October 26 the Ochsner trustees were informed that their bid was accepted and they might have access to the property to begin the conversion. The deal was completed on November 2.

On November 8, 1946, the foundation trustees chose a name for their new facility. It was to be called Foundation Hospital, a name reflecting a decision that profoundly affected the future of the Ochsner Institutions. The question was whether the hospital would be operated by the clinic, a partnership engaged in the private practice of medicine, or by the foundation, a nonprofit association dedicated to medical research, education, and charity. Although the purchase of the buildings and equipment from the government had been made by the foundation, there was no legal reason why the facility could not have been leased to the clinic for operation. The trustees decided, however, that if the clinic took over the hospital, it would appear that it was not to be run as a nonprofit institution, and this, in Guy Caldwell's words, "would constitute a breach of good faith." The trustees, anticipating the day when they would have to seek public contributions to build a permanent hospital, realized that their appeal would be weak if it were made on behalf of a private, profit-making partnership. It was a lesson that had been brought home to them early, when they had vainly sought help from foundations and philanthropists in financing the organization of the clinic.

The decision made on that Friday evening in 1946 was indeed to have far-reaching consequences. Because the foundation was recognized as a vital regional health resource in which the public has a stake, it was later possible to build and operate the present magnificent facility on Jefferson Highway. But in 1946 such a hospital as that was only a dream, and for all that the founders formally renamed Camp Plauché the Foundation Hospital, it was to be known to those who staffed it as Splinter Village.

CHAPTER FIVE

Splinter Village

The base hospital at Camp Plauché was an admirable setting for sick soldiers, men who were accustomed to spartan surroundings and no privacy at all. It would not have been the first choice of a society matron as the hospital in which to have a hysterectomy. The facility consisted of fifty-three frame buildings, connected by long, covered walkways. In each of the buildings where patients were housed, there were only two private rooms, one at each end. In converting the wards for civilian use, the Ochsner planners provided small cubicles with temporary partitions and curtains that could be drawn to keep personnel and visitors traversing the aisles from peeking in while physicians made physical examinations. More than one potential patient took one look around and walked out. Edgar J. Saux recalled the arrival of Gary Cooper, when he came to have his hernioplasty performed by Dr. Ochsner. "I met him at the airport," Saux related. "We wanted to give him as much privacy as we could, and when we arrived at the hospital I didn't take him to the regular entrance. We drove into the grounds. He had to walk through mud and then climb a rail to get into one of the walkways. He had a funny look on his face, but he didn't back out."

Mosquitoes were pesky. The summer sun beat down. Public transportation was inadequate, and the taxicab ride from downtown New Orleans, or even from the Prytania Street Ochsner Clinic, five miles away, was expensive. But many patients accepted the inconveniences in good spirit. After a few days they found kindred souls among their ward mates. A feeling of friendly concern developed. Everyone was in-

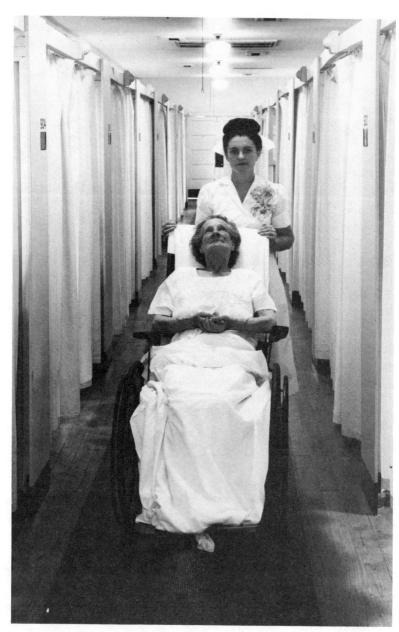

A ward in the Foundation Hospital

terested in the welfare of the patient in the next bed, and nurses and orderlies had all the volunteer help they could use.

For all its drawbacks, Splinter Village had the blessing of almost unlimited space. One of the old army wards became one of the nation's first recovery rooms, where highly trained nurses and technologists took patients from the operating tables and saw them through the critical early hours. And there was room for the patients' families, too. Surgeons noticed that members of the family often used to walk beside a patient's stretcher when he was being wheeled to the operating pavilion. Then they would go into a large empty room nearby to await the outcome. Somebody had the idea of staffing the room with an attendant and providing refreshments during the period of anxiety. It became routine for surgeons to make periodic visits to the room to keep relatives informed on the progress of the surgery, and the family lounge became an Ochsner's trademark.

The relatives who accompanied patients to Splinter Village also needed a place to sleep and eat, for many of them had traveled there from out of town, even out of the country. Some members of the medical staff and key laymen saw a business opportunity. They chartered the Orleans Service Corporation in 1946, and by the time the hospital opened early the next year they had accommodations ready. They created lodgings in some of the empty buildings of the former Camp Plauché post hospital and set up a cafeteria in another. Jefferson House, they called the project.

The corporation issued 280 shares of stock with a par value of $100 each. Of these shares, 70 were designated as Class A voting stock and were reserved for the seven trustees of the foundation. The other 210 shares were offered to staff doctors and the business manager, Junius Underwood. The trustees were designated as the board of directors, but they delegated the duties of running the operation to an advisory committee of the Class B nonvoting stockholders and never interfered in its workings.

The clinic, still located in the Physicians and Surgeons Building at Prytania and Aline streets, had purchased the nearby Briede home in 1945. At the same time it bought the vacant lot at St. Charles and Foucher, next door to the Briede residence. In 1948, the clinic arranged for the Orleans Service Corporation to take over this property, rent free, and operate it as a boardinghouse for out-of-town clinic patients.

When the new hospital was being planned in 1953 the foundation trustees knew that an adjacent hotel would be needed. The Orleans Service Corporation arranged to sell a new $350,000 stock issue to medical staff members and senior employees in order to complete the financing for a facility expected to cost $700,000. The new hotel was named Brent House in honor of Theodore Brent.

Over most of the years of its existence, the Orleans Service Corporation was profitable and paid good dividends to its shareholders, all of whom were partners or employees of the Ochsner institutions. When the enterprise faltered on one occasion, hotel consultant Olaf Lambert was brought in and quickly had the hotel making money again. In 1979 the trustees decided that Brent House would make a continuing source of revenue for the Foundation, and made a generous offer for all of the service corporation's stock. Shareholders agreed to sell. One doctor, who had purchased 1,500 shares for $15,000, was paid $160,000 for the 15,000 shares he then owned as the result of a ten-for-one stock split.

There was space at Splinter Village not only for the families of patients but for the families of staff members as well. As a fringe benefit, some members of the medical and administrative staffs were allowed to convert unused buildings to living quarters. They paid no rent and were given free utilities but had to bear the costs of turning bare structures into apartments. The grassy areas between the buildings became playgrounds, and the toddlers also could ride their tricycles down some of the long walkways. Along with the unusual hospital noises, patients could sometimes hear the happy sounds of children at play. Evelyn LeTard, wife of anesthesiologist Francis X. LeTard, remembers her family's years at Camp Plauché as an enjoyable period. In the Splinter Village doctors' colony were the families of Roswell D. Johnson, Harrison Snyder, William Spears Randall, George Bass Grant, and Dave Davis. Ada B. Anker, director of nursing services, lived there, as did Albert H. Scheidt, the hospital director, and Major Charles Holmes.

Out of the camaraderie that developed in Splinter Village, some of the doctors' wives developed a formal organization to foster social interaction. The Hospitality Club of the Ochsner Foundation was organized in 1954 at a meeting in the auditorium of the old hospital. "We are not a ladies' auxiliary in the usual sense," explained Evelyn LeTard, charter member, third president, and historian of the club. "We are a 'welcome wagon' group of staff wives who offer their services to new fellows and staff members and their families to help them become established and feel wanted." In addition to smoothing the transition for newcomers, the club stages periodic events at which doctors and their families mingle socially. Expressing his gratitude, Alton Ochsner wrote in 1969, "This is one of the things that makes this organization what it is."

The list of presidents reflects the name of many of the staff leaders. Serving, in order, were the wives of A. Seldon Mann, Edgar Little, LeTard, Thomas Weiss, Mercer Lynch, John Weed, Robert Lynch, William Arrowsmith, Herbert Christianson, Patrick Hanley, Don Samples, Joseph Bradford, James Fruthaler, John Jackson, John Holland, William Locke, Charles Moore, William Coleman, Gordon McFarland, Frank Riddick, Paul Murison, Chesley Hines, William Geary, Noel Mills, Luther C. Williams, William T. Mitchell, Harold Fuselier, Kenneth Bell, Robert J. Marino, Joseph Dalovisio, and David J. Elizardi.

The Foundation Hospital began its work on January 21, 1947, when the first four patients were admitted. The facility was like a dilapidated dump truck in which a Rolls-Royce engine had been installed. A high-powered staff was treating patients in third-rate surroundings. But in seven years at Splinter Village, the Ochsner Foundation learned how to run a hospital. And it was there that Ochsner began its pursuit of excellence, initiating traditions that still prevail. Despite the meager surroundings, for example, the trustees were determined that the food be of the highest quality. Dieticians were instructed to buy the best meat and produce and to cook meals with a tangy New Orleans flavor.

One of the patients who checked into the Foundation Hospital on opening day was Mrs. Halbert David Oakley, the wife of a dentist who practiced in Starkville, Mississippi. The following day, she became the first person to undergo surgery in the new facility. Curtis Tyrone performed the operation and reported its success to J. F. Eckford of Starkville, who had referred Mrs. Oakley to him. The hospital also received on opening day the first of many hundreds of patients from Latin

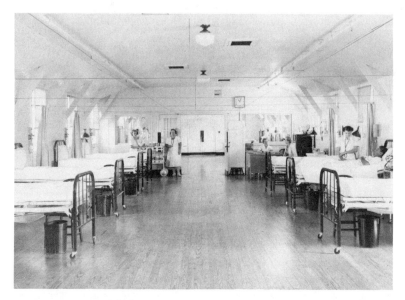

The intensive care unit at Splinter Village

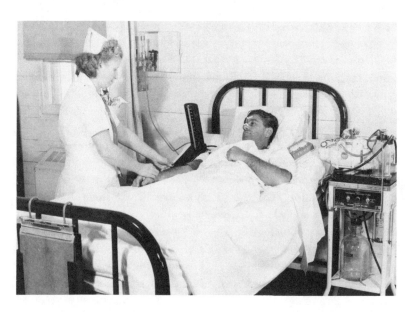

A blood pressure check in intensive care

America. Mercedes Melendez, seventy-five years old, of San Salvador, El Salvador, came in for removal of a lesion on her face. William Roland performed the surgery.

By the time dedication exercises were conducted on April 13, 1947, the training program for fellows had been approved by the American Medical Association and the American College of Surgeons. Forty-three residents were in that first class. Blanc Monroe, speaking at the ceremonies, said, "The basic rock upon which the Foundation rests is the determination to advance medical science and to relieve human suffering. Research, education and charity are the columns which support its rising arches. All people are to benefit physically, intellectually, and spiritually from its contacts. Any net profit to the Foundation must be applied to its educational charitable objects and none of it may be distributed to any individual under any circumstances." By that time, more than seven hundred patients had already been treated.

With per-bed costs averaging at least thirteen dollars a day, the new hospital was doomed to operate at a deficit at first. In addition to absorbing this deficit, the trustees also had to find a means of amortizing the $150,000 paid for the plant and $180,000 spent in conversion. The only likely source of funds was the clinic, on the rationalization that its income would increase because the staff would have beds for more patients. However, every dollar paid by the clinic to the foundation could only reduce the earnings of the partners, staff doctors, and employees. Nevertheless, the trustees—the same men who operated the clinic—concluded that the clinic would make the contribution. It was a commitment that would prove to be a heavy load in the years to come and would be regretted by the founders and the practitioners who came after them. Clinic doctors have paid their dues to the Ochsner Institutions.

Caldwell had hopes that the Veterans Administration and the Vocational Rehabilitation Department might share the expenses by using some of the Foundation Hospital facilities for an amputation center. The project did not develop, nor did a plan for using 75 to 150 beds for a crippled children's service.

And Splinter Village quickly developed into a headache for the foundation's trustees. "They opened too big," the clinic's business manager, Edgar J. Saux, explained many years afterward. "They had a waiting list of a couple of hundred patients for elective procedures, and the hospital was an instant success for about two weeks as these were admitted. Then the backlog ran out. The quickest way to lose your shirt is with an empty hospital. They finally had to close many beds." Patients complained of the noise and the cramped cubicles. Within a year of the dedication exercises, the problems of supporting the facility were so obvious and the future so questionable that staff and employee morale suffered. Caldwell felt a need to write a memorandum on March 19, 1948, saying rumors of an early closing of the hospital were unfounded. But months later, when the financial drain became a factor in staff unrest over salaries, the trustees did debate the advisability of shutting down the hospital.

The foundation had company in its travail. Dr. Odom's New Orleans Medical Foundation was sagging under the weight of a white elephant with a voracious appetite for money—the Lakeshore Hospital. It could be said that the Ochsner group had the last laugh, except that nobody saw anything funny about the situation. The New Orleans Foundation made overtures with a proposal that the two foundations operate one of the hospitals as a joint undertaking and close the other. Odom suggested that Lakeshore had better facilities, was more conveniently situated, and could be run more economically. But in a letter to Edgar Burns on October 13, 1948, Odom said if Ochsner refused the invitation, he would recommend that Lakeshore be abandoned and the staff send its patients to the Foundation Hospital.

Each group inspected the other's hospital. Afterward, Caldwell, who was almost never overridden by the other Ochsner founders, said it would be too expensive to transfer Foundation to Lakeshore and recommended that the Odom group move to Splinter Village under an arrangement that would permit its staff to maintain its separate identity. At a joint meeting of the two foundations on October 26, Caldwell and Burns ruled out any possibility that Ochsner would go to Lakeshore.

The private hospital operated by the New Orleans Medical Foundation went out of business the following spring when its lease on the site expired. The only medical facility then remaining on the prime lakefront acreage was the Musser-Gordon Hospital, conducted by the Charity Hospital administrators as a public facility for advanced tuberculosis patients. After Musser-Gordon ceased operation in late

1950 the area became a residential development. Ochsner thus outlasted the first hostile New Orleans group practice to challenge it in head-to-head competition, but there were reverberations later on. In 1958 Odom, as president of the Orleans Parish Medical Society, would block a proposal for the Ochsner staff to operate the independent service at Charity Hospital.

Nine months after Splinter Village opened, on September 19, 1947, the hospital staff encountered its first tropical storm. There was much apprehension as the blow approached, for nobody knew how the frame building of the hospital would withstand a pounding. As the winds grew in force, four of the staff doctors made their way to the scene. Alton Ochsner, Edgar Burns, Merrill Hines, and W. D. Davis circulated through the units, making themselves highly visible to reassure nervous patients. When the storm subsided, it was found that the hospital had come through with almost no damage, but at the supposedly more sturdy clinic building, Guy Caldwell and the maintenance crew had their hands full. Ochsner's and Burns's offices were flooded by rain pouring in through broken windows, and the files in the record room were also threatened. All had to be moved to a dry area. In addition, the clinic sheltered some thirty patients who had managed to get to the building in the expectation of fulfilling appointments. They took refuge in the lobby until they were able to escape during the lull that occurred while the eye of the storm was passing.

Although Splinter Village was the only hospital on the East Bank of Jefferson Parish, an area where traffic accidents were frequent, the founders were preoccupied with their goal of saving seriously ill patients who required tertiary care. They set up only minimal facilities for people who were injured or were felled by sudden illness. When the hospital first opened, the night nurse supervisor had to get a key and unlock the door to the emergency room whenever an after-hours patient sought attention. She also had to summon a house staff doctor from his regular duties to provide whatever services were needed.

The first emergency room was in the building closest to Jefferson Highway, where the blood bank and the equipment for electric shock treatment were also housed. Severely injured patients were treated in the surgery recovery room. After a year and a half, the emergency room was moved to the building next door, where heart catheteriza-

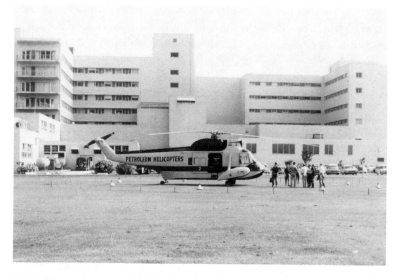

The first heliport at the new hospital

tion, proctoscopy, gastroscopy, and gynecologic examinations were also conducted. Even in the daytime, no physician was assigned full-time. The nurses called surgery whenever a patient appeared.

Thirty-five years later seven staff members, two fellows, and a crew of nurses and technicians are assigned to the fully equipped emergency suite on the ground floor of the hospital building to which Ochsner moved in 1954. In 1955 Ochsner's became the first hospital in the area to have a helicopter landing site on the grounds. Laura Howard and her son-in-law, Maurice Bayon, executive vice-president of Petroleum Helicopters, donated funds to provide the facility. Long ago the development of the industrial complex alongside the river between New Orleans and Baton Rouge, the burgeoning of offshore oil production in the Gulf of Mexico, and the population explosion made the emergency area one of the busiest on the campus.

The first crisis to test the ability of the new hospital to deal with disaster came on October 14, 1958. An explosion on an oil drilling platform twenty miles offshore took the lives of seven workers and injured a score of others. An hour and five minutes after the hospital received word of the blast, a helicopter landed with the first of nineteen men who were treated at Ochsner. Paul T. DeCamp, surgeon, who had attended a disaster course conducted by the American Hospital Association at Jacksonville, Florida, had set up a plan for handling a big influx of patients and had conducted a trial run. As a result, all nineteen men from the platform were treated within two hours, and all recovered. DeCamp's plan made it possible for the hospital to take care of as many as one hundred patients at a time and even to give emergency treatment to four hundred.

The emergency room was manned by the house staff on a rotating basis until 1964 when Charles E. Clark, who had just completed his residency in internal medicine, was made supervisor. In fourteen years on the assignment, Clark proved adept at meeting the special demands of emergency practice. The job calls for the ability to diagnose quickly and to deal with panicky patients. Clark also has the touch of a plastic surgeon in suturing cuts so that scarring will be minimal.

Clark's major challenge in the emergency room came in the aftermath of Hurricane Betsy, the first storm in history to result in property

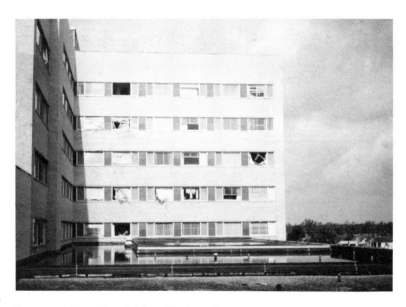

Damage to the new hospital from Hurricane Betsy

damage of more than a billion dollars, which hit New Orleans on September 9, 1965. He brought his wife and two children to the hospital as the storm approached and set them up overnight in the staff library while he awaited patients. On the night of the storm only eleven showed up. The next morning Clark walked outside and looked up at the higher floors of the wind-battered hospital. "I don't believe there was a single window unbroken," he relates. Rain had poured into the rooms with smashed windows, and the patients had to be rolled into the hallways to keep them dry. Clark recalled the mysterious disappearance of a large concrete block from the roof of the clinic building. "We guessed it must have blown away," he said.

Once the winds subsided, Clark and his associates were besieged by the greatest spate of patients ever to overrun the emergency room. For four or five days they came by the hundreds, lining the corridors while they awaited treatment of minor injuries such as glass in the eyes, cuts, and bruises. Others wanted typhoid vaccinations to protect them while they did relief work in flooded areas. The sleepless emergency room force kept on the job until all had been taken care of. As many as seven thousand received attention. Not a bill was mailed out by the hospital. "We certainly will not take advantage of a disaster like that," explained Mel Manning, administrative director.

The clinic took the same attitude in 1982 when a shutdown of the Kaiser Aluminum and Chemical Corporation plant in Chalmette threw hundreds out of work. Instead of sending bills to residents of the area, who might have been laid off, Ochsner wrote them letters inviting them to confer with clinic officials about arrangements that they would not find burdensome.

All personnel who deal with patients at a hospital know what it is to look tragedy in the face, but the emergency room workers must make the confrontation every day. Any ambulance that wheels up to the door may bring a child struck down by an automobile or a wage earner crippled in an industrial accident. The doctors and nurses steel themselves to do their jobs, but sometimes it is difficult to keep emotions under control. "The drownings were the worst," recalls Kathryn Oehlke, who served as a nurse in the Ochsner emergency service for seventeen years. "I dreaded having to face the family of a drowned child. Usually such a drowning occurs on a happy occasion, when they're on a family outing. Then it happens." She also cannot erase the memory of a distraught mother who let her child out of her car at school, then ran over him.

Once in a while, an incident lightens the tension. Clark tells of the father who brought in a small boy whose plastic toy automobile was lodged in his nose. "How in the world could he have done that?" the father wanted to know. Clark extracted the object and sent the pair home. Two hours later the father reappeared, with the toy embedded in *his* nose.

At 9:15 A.M. on Friday, June 22, 1979, the announcement over the loud speakers of "Code Red—Alert" put into motion a prearranged drill for the emergency mass casualties plan. At 9:30 the announcement of "Code Red—Activation" sent employees of key departments hurrying to their designated posts. Volunteers were taken to the physical therapy department as simulated victims of an industrial accident. When the drill was completed the announcement of "Code Red—All Clear" sent participants back to their regular duties. But two minutes later the emergency room received word that there had been an explosion and fire at a refinery at Norco, and injured persons were on their way to Ochsner. Again the "Code Red—Activation" signal was sounded, this time with the added announcement that it was no make-believe and had no connection with the drill. Thirty-three refinery employees were treated, most of them for chemical burns of the eyes.

The emergency room was also busy on the night when an airliner crashed into a hotel near the New Orleans International Airport killing or injuring many members of a high school class on a pregraduation tour. The crash of a chartered plane that was landing in a fog at the airport gave the emergency room crew another workout. But sometimes the finest emergency care is of no use. A disaster alert was put into effect when a ship struck and capsized a Mississippi River ferryboat at Luling, Louisiana. But it turned out that the emergency room was a quiet place that day. Almost all of the persons on the ferry were lost, not injured.

CHAPTER SIX

Weathering the Storm

Guy Caldwell wrote a memorandum on July 30, 1949, citing figures that seemed to vindicate the judgment of the founders in deciding to open a clinic geared to the medical needs of the Gulf South and areas of Latin America. By then, on average, seven thousand patients were seen every month. Significantly, a thousand of these were first-timers. Ninety percent came from the Gulf states, whereas Spanish-speaking Latin Americans made up a small but significant portion. The clinic staff had grown to sixty-two full-time and four part-time practitioners. Seventy fellows were being trained in nine specialties. Who could have guessed then that the Ochsner structure that seemed so solid was about to be buffeted by a storm that would shake its walls?

Yet the hurricane clouds were visible, especially to Caldwell. Of all the founders, he was best able to foresee threatening crises in the affairs of a center with a record of success that stirred envy in a competitive medical community. Within the next few years, decisions had to be made that would determine whether the phenomenon known as Ochsner would outlast the active careers of the Tulane professors or fade into oblivion upon the retirement or death of the five.

Most obviously, the need for permanent hospital accommodations for patients of the clinic staff had to be met. Splinter Village was a stopgap without any future and was available only on a temporary basis anyway. The founders still did not want to operate a hospital themselves, but they realized they needed one. Meanwhile, it was awkward and inefficient to have hospital and clinic separated by five miles of busy streets. Moreover, Splinter Village and the other activities of the foundation were straining the resources of the clinic to an extent never contemplated by the partners when they launched the foundation in 1944.

As vexing as the hospital and financial problems were, they had less potential long-term import than a situation that was surfacing in the professional staff. Employee-doctors began to find themselves underpaid. Many had several years of service invested in the clinic; yet there was no sign from above that the five founders had any idea of taking them into the partnership. Communications had broken down between founders and staff, and an exodus of the best qualified physicians became increasingly likely.

An account of how the conflicts were settled, how the need for hospital facilities was met, and how the clinic partnership evolved form a vital part of the story of the Ochsner Institutions. It makes no difference to a patient whether his doctor is a member of a partnership, whether he is paid a salary or a share of the revenues. But it is almost a matter of life or death whether his doctor practices in a disciplined environment where the standards of good medicine are enforced, where no ethical corner-cutting is permitted, where excellence is rewarded and failure punished. Good medicine started at Ochsner with the examples set by the founders and with the high levels they demanded of their employees. The eight years between 1949 and 1957 were pivotal in the history of the Ochsner Medical Institutions. Decisions made then set the New Orleans center on the road to its present eminence.

The Hospital

Soon after the first patients were admitted to the Foundation Hospital alongside the Huey P. Long Bridge, Guy Caldwell was already leading what would prove to be a frustrating quest for permanent access to beds. Even though the original three-year lease on Camp Plauché was later extended to nearly seven years, the founders had to race against time. They did not want to run a hospital. They tried again and again to work out arrangements to share the beds, operating rooms, and laboratories of another institution, but always they were thwarted, usually by unfriendly New Orleans doctors. In the long run, Ochsner benefited from the animosities; eventually, the founders had to swallow their qualms and begin building the campus on the Jefferson Highway. Without its ample facilities for treatment, research, and education—if Ochsner had been limited by the capacity of any other New Orleans medical center—it could not have lived up to its promise.

As early as 1944 Ochsner got a foretaste of the opposition that plagued all subsequent negotiations. A few weeks after it was chartered, the Ochsner Foundation asked the Touro administration to set aside ten beds for patients to be treated under the foundation's charity program. A committee of the Touro medical staff headed by James D. Rives intervened. Touro doctors were afraid that the foundation might eventually control the hospital's policies, forcing the independent staff doctors to practice elsewhere. They wanted to know what would become of Touro if Ochsner grew to tremendous size. The foundation trustees replied that "the proud history of Touro's 90 years refutes the implications that its board will ever be dominated by an outside influence." But the Touro board bowed to the wishes of the staff and refused to provide the beds.

Over a period of two years, 1946 and 1947, Caldwell and Maxwell E. Lapham, dean of the Tulane medical school, held a number of discussions looking toward a virtual merger of the foundation and the school. Tulane and the foundation would join forces in a public drive for funds to erect a three-hundred-bed university hospital, a new classroom building for the school, and a structure that would be leased to the Ochsner Clinic for use as its home base. The hospital would be operated by the foundation, and any deficit would be absorbed by the clinic. The hospital would be open to the patients of all Tulane faculty, whether or not the doctors were on the staff of the Ochsner Clinic. The board of trustees of the foundation would be increased to nine members, five representing the clinic and four from the board of administrators of Tulane.

Dean Lapham said the Tulane administrators would not approve any such plan unless full control of the foundation and its related activities were placed in their hands. Caldwell then suggested that Tulane operate the hospital and that the foundation contribute $60,000 a year toward the expenses. This arrangement also was rejected.

In 1948 Esmond Phelps, A. B. Freeman, and A. B. Paterson, Tulane administrators, proposed that Tulane, Ochsner, and Touro jointly solicit funds for the construction of a new wing at Touro with two hundred beds for Tulane faculty members, including those on the Ochsner staff. At a meeting on June 9, 1948, a committee was named to draw up a formal plan for the three-way affiliation. Caldwell was designated to represent Ochsner; John C. MacKenzie, Touro; and Lapham, Tulane. Blanc Monroe of Ochsner, Walter Barnett of Touro, and Esmond Phelps formed a legal committee to write a contract embodying any arrangement reached by the other committee. Within a month the Caldwell-MacKenzie-Lapham committee had produced a tentative agreement, and the lawyers began putting it into legal form. The proposal contemplated a $2 million addition that would increase the Touro capacity to 600 beds. There would be a Tulane unit of 350 beds for the Tulane staff, including Ochsner doctors, and a Touro unit of 250 beds for members not connected with Tulane.

The Touro staff made its feelings known at a meeting called for consideration of the proposition. Sixty doctors, half of them Tulane faculty members, voted unanimously against the affiliation. Eight Ochsner physicians, who also were present, did not vote. The Tulane professors who had no Ochsner connections made it clear they did not want to be part of a unit that included Ochsner men. They feared the arrangement would compel them to use Ochsner consultants, thus breaking up an unofficial combine of non-Ochsner faculty and independent Touro staff who referred patients to each other to the exclusion of Ochsner. In addition, the non-Tulane staff reasoned that a close-knit, well-organized Tulane unit would take over more and more beds, gradually displacing the Touro unit and eventually coming to dominate the hospital. Very obviously, the Ochsner Clinic was seen as an economic menace.

Other problems, in addition to staff opposition, contributed to the eventual abandonment of a three-way university hospital on the Touro grounds. The Touro board insisted it could not yield control of activities to outsiders. The Tulane administrators felt Touro could not reasonably expect Tulane to join in a drive for funds for a building at Touro and then leave all authority in the hands of the Touro board. Caldwell said the Ochsner group would not want to yield to the Touro board the sole responsibility for setting hospital fees. He noted that the infirmary, in keeping with philanthropist Judah Touro's will, charged private patients on a scale that provided support for the infirmary's charity services. The clinic objected to this arrangement, Caldwell said, because it was unfair to the paying patients. President Albert J. Wolfe said the Touro board would never give up its charity work, and he did not believe it would be possible to finance it solely with endowment funds.

At one point in the long-drawn-out negotiations, Rives reported that the Touro medical staff would not object to the construction of a wing at the infirmary to be leased to the Ochsner Foundation. But the staff wanted Tulane excluded from the arrangement. To this, the Ochsner trustees would not agree.

While Caldwell was dickering with Tulane and Touro, alternative possibilities arose. Although there was anti-Ochsner feeling among the medical staff at the Southern Baptist Hospital, Frank Trippe, the superintendent, told Caldwell that the Baptist trustees might be interested in building a separate unit for the clinic. But on August 16, 1949, Trippe informed Caldwell the trustees could not find money for the project and had therefore dropped the idea.

Opposition from the medical staff aborted discussions with the Sisters of Mercy, who were preparing to build the present facility of Mercy Hospital at Jefferson Davis Parkway and Bienville Street. Alton Ochsner talked with Archbishop Joseph F. Rummel, and reported the churchman "seemed extremely anxious that an affiliation be formed between the Clinic and a Catholic hospital." But this was not to be.

In four years of looking, Ochsner was never offered a firm commitment for the provision of 175 beds. Otherwise, the foundation would not have gone on alone. Edgar Burns had misgivings about the ability of the group to obtain the money to finance its own hospital. He raised the specter of losing access to Touro, having to close Splinter Village if the Illinois Central railroad refused to renew the lease, "and then having absolutely nowhere to place our patients." Francis LeJeune concurred. He was opposed to operating a hospital, for "as long as we carry the responsibility of the hospital, the Clinic will always be financially embarrassed by reason of deficits arising from hospital operation." Caldwell pointed out that if the foundation had to fall back on 125 beds that might be available at Touro, the average daily census of patients would be reduced by 50 beds. This, he said, would result in a loss of income to the clinic of at least $250,000 a year and would necessitate a 15 percent reduction in professional staff and lay personnel. The clinic would be set back to the situation that existed in 1947, when it either had to find enough beds or accept a limit on its possibility for growth.

On April 4, 1949, Caldwell wrote, "We can now assume that the negotiations between Touro and Tulane are at an end and have failed." By then, it was also obvious that Ochsner and Tulane could not reach agreement on the joint operation of a hospital. Burns earlier had summed up the feelings of the partners when he said that the "medical school will be in a position to dictate the number of beds that we can use, the kind of service to be given our patients, the number of fellows we can keep in training, and many other things which could cause embarrassment and lead to financial difficulties." And on June 18, 1949, Caldwell telephoned Wolfe on behalf of the Ochsner group to reject Touro's latest proposals. One was to provide 125 beds, an insufficient number, Caldwell explained. And the other was for Ochsner alone to raise $750,000 to finance 75 additional beds, which, added to the 125 offered by Touro, would make the 200 beds the clinic wanted. "We cannot accept the entire responsibility for providing all the funds needed for additional beds," Caldwell said.

During the following year there would be revivals of hope of affiliation with Baptist or Mercy. Officials of the Episcopal diocese of Louisiana discussed the feasibility of building a hospital and expressed great interest in affiliating it with the Ochsner Foundation. Guy Caldwell told Bishop Girault M. Jones the foundation would supply a list of likely donors to help the Episcopalians in a fund drive. He also asked Jesse Bankston of the state hospital board to give special consideration to any Episcopal application for state aid. But the diocese soon decided the undertaking was too large.

None of these glimmers of hope raised in 1950 amounted to much. Essentially, by spring, 1949, the foundation trustees had resigned themselves to the conclusion that their hospital would have to be a do-it-yourself project. And they were determined that the entire cost be paid from public contributions and from any available government funds. Caldwell set forth the trustees' sentiments when he wrote that the "foundation should insist that hospital be fully paid for by donations because it is unfair and poor business to charge a profit for medical care in Clinic and Hospital, sufficient to amortize large indebtedness. The cost of medical care alone, with reasonable salaries and security for physicians and other personnel serving them and support of the Fellowship Program, is all that should be taken from patients, whether in the Clinic or in the Hospital."

If a date were to be chosen for the conception of the present home of the Ochsner Medical Institutions, it most logically would be July 25, 1949. At a meeting on that day the foundation trustees asked Dr. Ochsner to consult Raymond T. Rich Associates about the possibilities of a campaign for public donations for a new hospital. Ochsner conferred with Rich in New York and learned that a pilot study could be made for $1,500. Thomas Devine, Rich's associate, came to New Orleans for a discussion with the trustees.

Several factors would make fund raising difficult. Guy Caldwell pointed out two of the biggest obstacles in a memorandum:

> Because of the rather spectacular growth of the Clinic and Foundation that is self-evident to the Community and patients, and because this has been accomplished without publicity or any appeal for financial support, the prevailing opinion is that Clinic and Foundation are private money-making concerns with huge income, quite adequate to finance their own expansions and do not require any public assistance. In a vague way the Community is glad to have the Clinic and regards it as something of an asset, but there is no sense of obligation to support the Foundation's programs of education, research and charity.
>
> The medical profession of New Orleans and the surrounding country opposed the organization of the Clinic and a large part is still very antagonistic to its development, although admitting that the Clinic is strictly ethical, does good work and that its activities really supplement rather than interfere with their practices. The anti-clinic group encourages the public's feeling that the Clinic and Foundation are rich and amply able to finance their own projects for expansion.

The very name, Alton Ochsner Medical Foundation, was a handicap, according to Raymond Rich, because in the public mind foundations were wealthy associations that donated money; they did not ask for it. Moreover, the organization of the Ochsner institutions was confusing to outsiders, who did not perceive the difference between clinic and foundation. Prospective donors might think they would only be adding to the incomes of practitioners who were already earning what the public would consider good salaries.

Nevertheless, the Rich organization believed a preliminary study would be of value, and the trustees agreed. In the summer of 1949 the firm conducted a three-month pilot study to determine the probable public reaction to a fund-raising drive. The final report recommended that the clinic take steps to bolster staff morale and that the foundation conduct a public information program stressing its research and education activities. If these two things were done, the Rich firm foresaw a successful campaign. On November 29, 1949, the trustees voted a $36,000 appropriation for a year-long campaign. On March 31, 1950, they signed an agreement with Raymond Rich Associates to direct the effort. The goal was $4 million, and no one expected the contributions to come flooding in.

Sites

Even before the founders concluded they would have to build their own facility, they were on the lookout for a suitable site. Foundation Hospital might have been built on the New Orleans lakefront. It might have been on Park Island, now a posh residential enclave on Bayou St. John across from City Park—or it could have been in the park itself. It could have occupied the site of the old Pelican Stadium at Carrollton and Tulane avenues. It could have arisen on the tree-shaded property of the Poydras Home for Elderly Ladies in the 5300 block of Magazine Street. These and numerous other locations were considered during a four-year hunt that ended with the purchase of the Riding Academy site. From the upper floors of the high-rise clinic, hospital, and Brent House buildings, and from the parking garage, patients have a sweeping view of the Mississippi River from Audubon Park past the Huey P. Long Bridge to the west bank beyond the Avondale Shipyard. The never-ending parade of tankers, freighters, and barge tows reminds onlookers that they are viewing one of the nation's busiest seaports.

Stanley M. Lemarie, who negotiated the purchase of the first clinic properties in the Touro Infirmary area, and the real estate developer Allen H. Johness offered prospective locations to the trustees. Johness' list included a tract near Carrollton Avenue opposite the Catholic archdiocese property on Walmsley Street, a site on Stroetlitz Street for which $145,000 was asked, and the area bounded by Dante, General Ogden, Palmetto, and Edinburgh streets in the neighborhood of the present Carrollton Shopping Center. He also suggested the Pelican baseball field at Carrollton and Tulane avenues, now occupied by the Fountain Bay Hotel. Lemarie came up with the seven-and-one-half-acre Park Island and an adjacent area bound by Bancroft Drive, Mirabeau, Cartier, and Fillmore streets. He also proposed two sites near the New Basin Canal, which had not then been filled, one on West End Boulevard, and another on Pontchartrain Boulevard. Lemarie and Curtis LeJeune even talked with Mayor de Lesseps S. Morrison about the possibility of acquiring space in an unused portion of City Park.

A tract comprising five city blocks in the area where the Lakeshore Hospital was being phased out was rejected because of the $400,000 price tag. The campus of the Baptist Bible Institute on Washington Avenue, where Newcomb College once was situated, was ruled not suitable because the buildings could not readily be converted to hospital use. Administrators of the Poydras Home talked of selling the Magazine Street property to Ochsner, then changed their minds. The trustees rejected a location near Hotel Dieu because they believed the area was deteriorating. A forty-acre tract at Southport, on the river near the Orleans-Jefferson parish boundary and only a few blocks from the present campus, won temporary favor, and the trustees briefly eyed the site of the old dog-racing track on Jefferson Highway at Shrewsbury Road, between Splinter Village and the present hospital. But when the fund-raising campaign began, no site had yet been chosen.

The Campaign Begins

To use a Wall Street expression, the Alton Ochsner Medical Foundation "went public" in 1950. The history of many an American enterprise includes the same chapter: Entrepreneurs with a salable idea open a business on a shoestring, with their own funds. It thrives. The time comes when the opportunity for expansion beckons, but an infusion of cash far beyond the company's resources is needed. The solution is to bring in new capital by selling stock to the public. A private firm develops into a great corporation.

During the first years after 1944 the foundation's educational, research, and charitable functions had been supported by the Ochsner Clinic and by sporadic gifts from individuals and pharmaceutical companies. It was clear that the clinic, entering the most difficult months of its existence because of staff unrest, could not shoulder the burden of financing a new hospital. Its resources were extended to the limit by Splinter Village, and the founders had had to borrow money to keep that facility open. The only alternative was to ask the public to underwrite the cost of building a hospital and maintaining the foundation's research, educational, and charitable programs. But could the residents of the Gulf South be persuaded to dip into their bank accounts to subsidize this medical court of last resort, this institution where young doctors could get first-class graduate training, this setting of laboratories where scientists were working on the cures for disease? The founders were not sure of the answer.

In going public with the opening of the fund drive in the spring of 1950, the Ochsner Foundation had no stock to offer, of course. What it sold was a concept. Once the doctors appealed to the public for financial help in making their dream come true, they shared their ownership with those who responded, and many did respond.

The most generous supporters of the Ochsner Medical Institutions over the years have been members of the family of the late L. O. Crosby, Sr., founder of a lumber and chemical empire headquartered in Picayune, Mississippi, and De Ridder, Louisiana. Their gifts and bequests will total more than $6.5 million. Donors have included Mrs. Dorothy Crosby, Mrs. Hollis H. Crosby, L. O. Crosby, Jr., L. O. Crosby III, Mr. and Mrs. R. Howell Crosby, Ethel Crosby, and Crosby companies and foundations.

Certainly, the Crosbys were not the only benefactors. Ben Hogan, remembering how Alton Ochsner's skill had saved his life, volunteered his time and his name as general chairman. Rudolph Matas, then in his ninetieth year, served as honorary chairman. In addition, whatever the attitude of the rest of the medical profession had been, the lay community in and around New Orleans had come to respect the Ochsner Institutions, and that community could easily see the need for more hospital beds. In one year, contributions and pledges from the local area reached $962,000.

Even the mayor of New Orleans, deLesseps S. Morrison, took an interest in the campaign, particularly when rumor reached him that Houston was trying to lure the Ochsner Institutions away from New Orleans. On July 6, 1950, Morrison addressed a letter to Alton Ochsner, who was away on a trip to Spain.

> It has come to the attention of this office that the city of Houston has displayed considerable interest in having you establish your clinic in that city. This news has perturbed us here in New Orleans greatly, and I am writing this letter to prevail upon you, that before you make any final decision regarding the site of the Ochsner Clinic, that we in New Orleans be given an opportunity to discuss plans at length with you.
>
> The Ochsner Clinic has served an excellent purpose and is definitely a community lead here in New Orleans, and we sincerely hope that the news of a possible transfer to Houston is merely rumor and that you will continue to maintain your clinic here in New Orleans.

The mayor's news was more fact than rumor. The Texas city, on its way to becoming the largest metropolis in the South, had begun to pull together the elements that have made it a world-famous medical center. Addition of the renowned Ochsner Clinic to the complex of hospitals and university facilities would have been a civic coup. Ochsner officials had indeed been talking with Houstonians, including Dr. E. W. Bertner, president of the Texas Medical Center, and Frank C. Smith, president of the Houston Natural Gas Association. And although the discussions were informal, their undertone was serious.

On July 26, Caldwell thanked Mayor Morrison on behalf of Ochsner, who was still in Europe. "All of us," he wrote, "have been deeply gratified, both by the tribute Houston has paid to our work and by the interest of New Orleans people in our remaining here. Of course we feel that New Orleans is our home and we want to stay here. We are doing everything in our power to work out a plan of replacing the present inadequate Foundation Hospital with a new, modern hospital building, suitable for specialized surgery and treatment, for the program of specialists' training, and for research work." The New Orleans Commission Council responded by adopting a resolution endorsing the campaign for funds to build the present Ochsner campus, and thoughts of taking the clinic to Houston died out.

Outside of New Orleans, however, the going was harder. In community after community, Rich's campaign workers ran into hostility among local practitioners who opposed what they called "building up the Ochsner crowd." Rich attributed this attitude to a fear that, as the Ochsner fame spread, the doctors would lose their more affluent patients to the New Orleans center. His initial approach was to organize a committee of laymen and physicians in each town to spearhead the campaign. Almost invariably, the organizer was asked why residents outside of New Orleans should contribute to building a New Orleans hospital. The explanation that the South needed its own facility for the treatment of difficult cases and for research and training usually brought a positive response.

Opposition from doctors was subtle in most communities; usually, local practitioners simply suggested that charity begins at home and that local hospital facilities were needed. Doctors who had trained at the Foundation Hospital gladly campaigned for what they referred to as the "Mayo of the South." Yet in most cities, friendly physicians, pleading that they had to get along with their fellow practitioners, offered to help raise money only if they could remain in the background.

In Jackson, Mississippi, physicians conducted a counter campaign against Ochsner. They called on prospective donors to discourage them from giving to the New Orleans center. They even organized a drive for funds for a local hospital after Ochsner organizers had come to town. The pressure forced one Jackson physician to drop out as cochairman of an Ochsner dinner after the affair had been scheduled.

In the face of such hostility, Rich's organizers found it increasingly difficult to recruit committee members. In towns where committees had started off with a burst of enthusiasm, some ceased to function, despite prodding. There were exceptions to this pattern. In Shreveport, for example, a group of leading citizens continued to be highly productive. Nevertheless, by the end of the first year of fund raising, Rich's local committee system had all but collapsed.

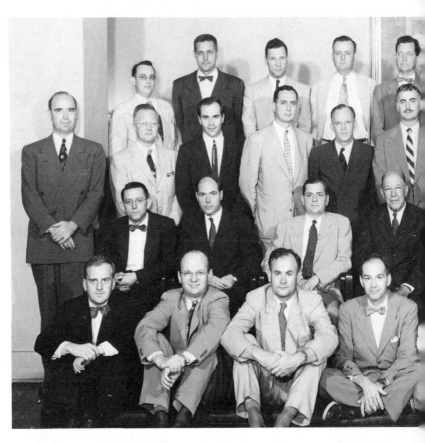

Some of the members of the Foundation Hospital staff in May, 1953. *Back row, left to right*: Clarence Black, Thomas Lee Duncan, E. Leland Eggleston, R. Jocelyn Crawley, John C. Weed, Robert Birchall, Arthur M. Blood, Martin J. Bechtol, Thomas E. Weiss, and Malcolm B. Burris; *second row from back*: Homer D. Kirgis, Harold Horack, David D. Vaughan, Harold V. Cummins, William R. Arrowsmith, Walter Culpepper, Gustave Fred Weber, Mary Sherman, Frederick W. Brewer, George E. Beckman, Jr., and

The Clinic Staff Rebels

For the first seven and a half years, the clinic was operated as the private fiefdom of the founding partners, who had, after all, taken the financial risks involved, drawn salaries considerably smaller than each could have earned in private practice, and made substantial donations that put the foundation on its feet. They may have remembered Frank Lahey's exhortation to keep tight controls and run the clinic them-

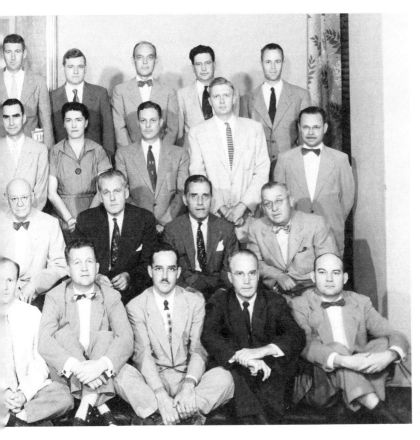

Lester L. Weissmiller; *third row from back*: Vincent Derbes, Otto Schales, Rawley M. Penick, Jr., Charles Eshleman, Mims Gage, Willoughby E. Kittredge, Thomas Findley, and George Bass Grant; *front row*: William Locke, Merrill O. Hines, George Schneider, C. Harrison Snyder, Roger D. Bost, Francis X. LeTard, Paul T. DeCamp, Dean H. Echols, and Charles Jackson Ray

Leon Trice Photography

selves, although none needed this advice. Every one of the five was a stubborn, forceful individualist accustomed to making his own decisions.

In the first few years, appointments to the salaried staff in the flourishing clinic were prized, especially by doctors being discharged from the armed services who had no established practices of their own to come home to. It was comfortable to be a member of a group, relieved of such onerous aspects of solo practice as collecting bills, meeting payrolls, answering nighttime and weekend emergency calls. Because the clinic stressed tertiary care by specialists and offered a full schedule of challenging cases to its staff, the founders were able to recruit talented employee-doctors, many of whom lived up to their promise and established national reputations of their own.

Yet, the founders came up in an era when interns and residents worked for room and board and little more, when senior practitioners lorded it over junior colleagues. They were not conditioned to be sensitive to the feelings of hired doctors. They also were busy with their own patients, and they were enjoying the rewards of their own career successes. Although the senior members of the hired medical staff were their professional peers, the partners issued orders without consulting them. Instructions came in the form of ukases. A wall divided proprietors from the hired help. Admittedly, not one of the original partners, not even Guy Caldwell, would have qualified as the personnel director of a corporation.

Even so, had there been better communications, the staff uprising might never have occurred; at least its acrimony would have been avoided. Early on, as Caldwell's memoranda and the minutes of meetings make clear, the founders were aware that staff members would eventually have to be rewarded with some kind of participation in the ownership of the clinic. But the employee-doctors did not know this, and many felt they were being exploited. They might have been more patient had they been told a solution was being considered. In summing up the status of clinic and foundation on July 25, 1949, for example, Caldwell wrote that any provision for future ownership would have to take note of the claims of the others. "Many of the senior members on our staff feel that it is due them to establish a plan for succession which will give them some assurance that the transitional stage will not be too critical, and that as some of them prove their administrative ability, they will soon begin to have some voice in the policies and plans for the Clinic. Those who have given five to eight years of loyal service to the group are due some clarification of this problem before long."

The gentle Julie Wilson composed what may be described as the staff's Magna Carta in the same month. It was a conciliatory document, but even so, it led to a breakthrough that resulted in today's self-

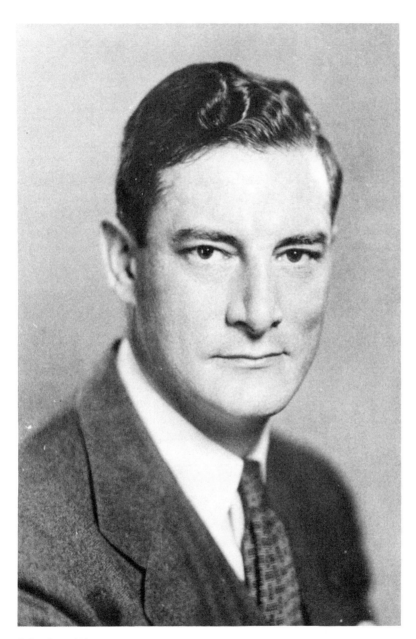

Julius Lane Wilson

governing medical staff. Wilson noted that he, as director of the clinic, and Dean Echols, as director of education for the foundation, provided some input from the doctor-employees at partner meetings, "but the staff has no direct means of expressing its natural interest in the operation of the Clinic. Moreover, it would be desirable to have certain members of the staff gain some experience in the administration of the Clinic." He hastened to add that he did not propose that finances be discussed with staff representatives. The founders would have been appalled at such a thought. He suggested the formation of an administrative advisory committee, the members of which would be appointed by the partners for specific terms. The committee would advise the partners and also would act as a conduit between the staff and the clinic owners. Try out the plan for two years, he suggested. If it proved effective, the committee could then take over administrative functions, exclusive of finances.

On August 2, 1949, the partners approved Wilson's suggestion, and appointed six staff doctors—Thomas Findley, Dean Echols, T. L. L. Soniat, John Weed, Edgar Little, and Willoughby Kittredge—to the administrative advisory committee for one-year terms. Many years later Kittredge, the first chairman, said that the founders had accepted a committee only because "they wanted somebody to share the blame," that they regarded it as window dressing. As a matter of fact, the founders did pay scant attention to their advisors for nearly a year.

The founders themselves had been dissatisfied with their partnership agreement almost from the beginning. They had considered changing it either into an association similar to the one that operated the Mayo Clinic or into a foundation of the type governing the Cleveland Clinic and the Ford Hospital. But Monroe informed the partners that state law forbade the practice of medicine by a nonprofit corporation. He furthermore questioned the advisability of converting the partnership into an association. In 1949 Monroe conceded that it might by then be legal for a foundation to engage in the practice of medicine in Louisiana. He agreed that from the standpoint of public relations and taxation, it might be ideal to put all activities under the foundation's control. But he continued to block any change. He was afraid that the Treasury Department would go to Congress for legislation outlawing such an arrangement. Furthermore, he felt that the foundation plan

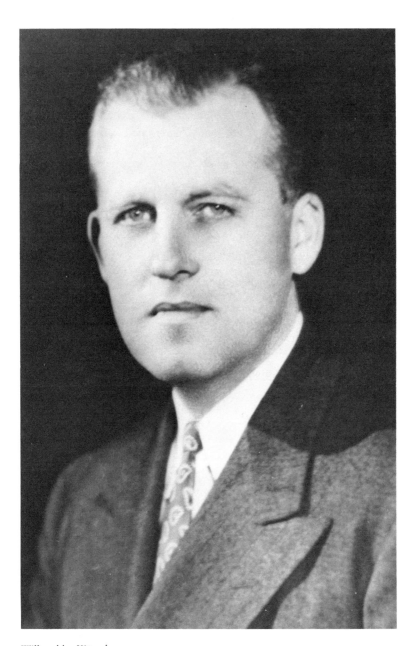

Willoughby Kittredge

would be opposed by the Orleans Parish Medical Society, and enough political pressure might be generated in the legislature to prohibit it by state law. Although Theodore Brent, leaning toward the partners, questioned whether public sentiment would support legislation aimed at the foundation, the clinic and the foundation continue today as separate entities. It is a measure of the influence exerted by J. Blanc Monroe on the development of the Ochsner Medical Institutions.

As 1950 began, Guy Caldwell addressed his concerns about the clinic-foundation relationship to Monroe. He and the other partners, along with a majority of the staff, believed the activities of the foundation had "drained the Clinic of its financial resources to a dangerous extent." Monroe's idealistic concept of the foundation as a vehicle "to advance medical science and to relieve human suffering" had collided with the economic realities facing those who had to pay most of the bill. Except for the income from hospital services, the clinic was the foundation's only means of support and therefore was financially squeezed. The "majority of Staff members are convinced that their salaries are inadequate to meet their living expenses and obligations and that Partners have no right to persist in a policy that robs them of their just dues over a prolonged period of time," Caldwell informed the attorney. "They would like to see all donations of the Partnership to Foundation eliminated and the same amount used to augment their salaries. If no other way can be provided for maintaining Foundation activities, it would be only fair to take this step."

The financial plight was real. When the hospital was opened in 1947, the foundation was able to borrow money to finance the facility only because the clinic pledged itself to cover any operating deficit. Transactions between clinic and foundation were governed by restrictions imposed by the Internal Revenue Service. The clinic was allowed to donate 15 percent of its pretax profits, and it also paid one dollar a day as a credit for each hospital bed. By 1951 the clinic had been subsidizing the foundation at a rate of more than $100,000 per year. In the spring of 1950, the clinic owed the Hibernia Bank $272,000, for which the founders were personally responsible.

By the time the founders had reluctantly concluded in early 1950 that they would have to build their own hospital, Rich Associates found the staff mutinous; morale was on the skids largely because of inadequate salaries. Obviously, the founders would have to tidy up their home base before striking out into new territory. Rich urgently recommended higher incomes for the staff even in the face of declining revenues. He suggested that expenses be held to the minimum and that the doctors be promised a 10 percent bonus at the end of the fiscal year, on April 30, 1950, to augment small salary increases for those who had been on the staff two years or longer.

Circumstances had at last forced the hand of the partners. They summoned the members of the administrative advisory committee, along with Raymond Rich, his associate Thomas Devine, and Julius Wilson, into what amounted to an emergency meeting on April 11, 1950. The partners were finally looking for support for the staff, and they turned to the committee.

Alton Ochsner began the meeting by conceding that months had passed without any input being asked of the committee, but from now on, he told the group, the advice of its members would be sought. Caldwell then took the floor and described the appointment of the committee as a definite move for staff participation in policy making. He explained Rich's suggested bonus plan and informed the committee members that they, as the representatives of the staff, could make a decision that would be binding on the other doctors. The five partners, he said, would not share in the proposed bonus but would continue at the same level of income even though they had not increased their drawings for several years. Caldwell also explained the background of the decision to build an Ochsner hospital and solicited the committee's support in the drive for funds.

When Caldwell had finished his remarks, the committee voted unanimously in favor of the bonus plan. Two or three members suggested that the partners should also benefit from the bonus, but Duke Le-Jeune said that since net earnings would not be large during the fiscal year, the partners would pass this time. The committee also undertook to enlist the support of the other staff doctors in the hospital fund raising.

The first glimmerings of staff democracy had penetrated the closed councils. Troubles and conflicts lay ahead, and seven years would elapse before employee-doctors gained a foothold into the ownership. In retrospect, the dictatorial control of the founders in the early days seems to have served a purpose. They were perfectionists in their own practices, demanded expert medicine from the physicians and surgeons on the staff, and had the authority to enforce their decisions. They set standards that subsequent generations would strive to maintain.

The outbreak of the Korean War in June, 1950, was followed by a sag in business activities, a condition always reflected in the revenues of medical institutions. In 1950 the clinic had 8,136 fewer patient registrations than in 1947, and the number of new patients fell by 2,091. The occupancy rate at Foundation Hospital was nearly forty patients per-day fewer in 1950 than in 1947.

Caldwell noted the depressing effect of the Korean conflict, but he added, "It now seems probable that the basic reason for the decreased volume of work has been the considerable increase in the number of doctors and competent specialists who have established themselves in the smaller centers throughout our drawing territory. Hospital facilities also have been improved in many of these places, whereas our Foundation Hospital is still very uninviting." Ochsner was only beginning to feel the effects of a boom in medical practice in the South that started after World War II and built steadily through the later 1950s, the 1960s, and the early 1970s. New or enlarged medical schools turned out doctors in numbers not dreamed of in the days before health insurance and governmental programs enabled practitioners to earn good livings. No longer did specialists congregate in a few cities. In short, the clinic and hospital at New Orleans now had competition, and they were suffering financially as never before.

The spring of 1951 brought the most serious crisis ever to threaten the continued existence of the organization. Staff unrest was boiling to the point of revolt. Low pay and uncertainty over the future began to produce the long-threatened exodus of valuable physicians. Afterward, Merrill Hines counted no fewer than thirteen men who quit in the period 1950–1952. In the month of June, 1951, alone, seven doctors either left or announced their intention of leaving. The clinic received a particularly bad blow when two gastroenterologists resigned, leaving nobody in that department. All the resignations presented serious problems for the clinic. Later, the mere rumor that Thomas Findley intended to leave and that Lodwick S. Meriwether planned to take five other internists from the staff to set up a private practice in Jackson, Mississippi, would produce prompt action from the board of administrators. According to Caldwell, the loss of that many men from the medical department would have reduced the clinic's work by 25 to 30 percent.

The exodus was also detrimental to the fund-raising drive. Raymond T. Rich and Associates reported that the resignations had removed "most of the chronic malcontents" but added that it would be extremely unfortunate to put all of those who had departed in that category.

> The departing doctors include a number with high professional stature. In the aggregate a considerable amount of professional prestige has been lost. . . . More important, however, is the fact that many of the doctors who left are unnecessarily bitter. The technique of speeding the departing staff member is even more important than the technique of welcoming a new associate. This is particularly true of a Clinic, the business of which is so largely dependent upon referrals. Regardless of the improvements, the morale of the staff is still not good. It would be unjust and cynical to attribute this solely to dissatisfaction over salaries. Some of the most loyal and enthusiastic believers in the Clinic feel that they have lost the sense of high adventure with which they and other members joined the staff some years ago. Part of the value of the executive committee is lost, simply because the staff does not know what the executive committee is doing and how it is functioning.

A happy staff could prove an invaluable fund-raising tool. On the other hand, discontented people or embittered former staff members would not be likely to persuade the public to support the Ochsner Institutions.

But there was no money for salary increases or bonuses for the physicians and surgeons who had cast their lots with the clinic and now found themselves earning less than their medical school classmates who had chosen solo practice. It was a talented group, chosen by the founders themselves as worthy future successors. These were the second generation, who in time would build on the framework established by the five Tulane professors and see the Ochsner Institutions solidify their national and international stature. They would win honors, including national presidencies, that would approach the achievements of the founders themselves. In 1951, however, they needed income more than they needed encomiums.

When the financial troubles of both clinic and hospital required negotiation of a loan from the Hibernia National Bank, Monroe, Brent, and George E. Conroy, managing partner in the New Orleans office of Haskins and Sells, auditors, had sharp words for the business decisions of the partners. They said retrenchments promised to the bank had not been put into effect in the first quarter of 1951. On the contrary, the three reported, expenditures during the quarter, including the partners' withdrawals, had been substantially greater, and no appreciable reduction in staff had been accomplished. As a matter of fact, they understood, "four more members of the staff were added in January." The three recommended a drastic cut in the salary load, dismissal of certain staff members, economies in the fellowship program, closure of units at the hospital, and the establishment of a committee that would control all expenditures and financial policies of the clinic. The partners agreed to cede financial control to a committee that included Monroe, Brent, and Hiram Kostmayer, the medical director. Moving to cut costs by $100,000 in the 1951–1952 fiscal year, the committee ruled out the replacement of staff doctors who had resigned, reduced the drawings of the partners, and eliminated expenditures for travel and entertainment.

At a later meeting the beleaguered partners suggested further consideration of closing the hospital, reorganizing the clinic, and curtailing its commitments to the foundation. On May 3 the partners adopted a resolution calling for drastic action. "Resolved that the Partnership is convinced that even after complete implementation of the suggestions of the Executive Committee the Clinic will continue bankrupt unless completely relieved of all obligations to Foundation except rental for Clinic buildings and facilities. Resolved further that Clinic must be relieved, as of May 1st, 1951, of all support of Foundation, specifically bed credits, contributions to Research, payment of deficits to Foundation Hospital and support of the post-graduate education program." They were barely talked out of closing the Foundation Hospital, a move that would have been enormously costly in the loss of public prestige.

At eight o'clock on the evening of May 9, 1951, Merrill Hines, president of the Foundation Hospital staff, called to order a meeting at which the disgruntled physicians and surgeons put their demands on the record. The partners were present at the start. Kostmayer discussed the financial problems and announced the dictates of his committee—all bad news. He said that because fees were higher, the clinic had collected only $56,000 less for professional services in 1950 than it had in 1947. But the clinic had added eleven doctors, and the salary budget was 50 percent higher. By prearrangement, the partners and Kostmayer then departed, and the fireworks started.

Dean Echols took the floor for twenty minutes. He said the clinic was in bad financial shape for many reasons. He conceded that the partners had taken a terrific beating financially, emotionally, and physically in their attempts to build a great clinic. Echols thought the Monroe-Brent-Kostmayer committee would balance the clinic budget but said the result would be bankruptcy of the physician employees. "Mr. Monroe and Mr. Brent are chiefly concerned with the development of a great scientific and educational foundation," Echols went on. "They are well on their way to success." He said part of their task was to raise money for the foundation, "and they are duty bound to obtain as much of the Clinic's income as possible."

Echols reminded the doctors that there had been no bonus for the staff in the previous fiscal year and that now benefits had been reduced by the elimination of travel and entertainment allowances. The time had come, he said, for staff members to stop complaining and looking elsewhere for jobs. Now they should petition the executive committee and the foundation trustees for a 10 percent salary increase retroactive to May 1; for a further 10 percent increase in the total salary budget on May 1, 1952, the money to be distributed as decided by the administrators; and for a sweetening of the retirement plan.

The neurosurgeon suggested the proposed higher salaries could be financed if the foundation would waive building rentals and hospital bed credits for the time being. "I was one of the promoters of the Foundation's educational, research and hospital programs," he recalled. "But I no longer can stand idly by and let the Foundation kill the goose that is laying the golden egg." He forecast that the foundation eventually would be rich and influential but said the clinic had contributed as much as it could at the time. Echols emphasized that he wanted no one to construe his stand as being one of "disloyalty, rebellion or unionism."

Without dissenting vote, the staff elected Echols and Julius Lane Wilson cochairmen of a committee to put Echols' suggestions into writing in a document to be signed by all members at a special meeting. A parade of speakers—including Paul T. DeCamp, Malcolm Burris, Rudolph M. Landry, Willoughby E. Kittredge, Mims Gage, Wilson, Jason Collins, A. J. Ochsner, John Weed, Mercer Lynch, Robert Birchall, and Walter Trautman—rose to endorse Echols' ideas. Most obviously, the doctors were not being stampeded by any cabal of revolutionaries.

But Blanc Monroe refused to yield. It would, he said, be utterly impossible for the clinic to meet the salary demands, which he insisted were not justified. After all, each founder had voluntarily decreased his draw during the 1951–1952 fiscal year by $3,000. In any case, Monroe believed, increases would be illegal under wartime regulations of the Treasury Department, an opinion in which Conroy, the auditor-advisor, concurred. Monroe lectured the partners on their obligations, pointing out that they had agreed to support the foundation and had obligated themselves for bank loans. Any change in the relationship between clinic and foundation would necessitate renegotiation of loans from the Hibernia Bank. Closing the Foundation Hospital would destroy its value as a going concern, would inflict a severe blow to the repute of the Ochsner doctors, and would force the dismissal of valuable personnel. Monroe would agree only to help formulate some plan for staff participation in policy making and then only if final control were left with the partners.

On one point, partners and staff were united: They wanted the institutions revamped immediately into some form of association or foundation that would operate clinic, hospital, and educational and research activities. Their thought was to have the governing organization pay salaries to partners and staff and to halt the subsidies to the foundation. They insisted this plan would allow salaries to become more equitable with the incomes of private practitioners. But against the influence of Monroe, even the potent combination of founders and staff could not prevail.

The first concrete proposal for bringing senior staff members into the ownership of the clinic came from the administrative advisory committee on May 28, 1951. Although the committee acknowledged the flaws in its plan, the arrangements suggested were not too different from those finally adopted in 1957 when the partnership was finally expanded. Highlights of the committee's plan were:

* On an appropriate date, such as December 31, 1951, the original partnership would be terminated. The five founders would divide all assets except the name and good will. (The clinic's main assets, as is true today, were accounts receivable. All property and equipment were, and are, leased from the foundation.)
* On the following day, control of the group practice would be transferred to an association made up of the five original partners and twenty-five of the senior staff doctors.
* The five original partners would come into membership in the association without paying for their shares. The twenty-five other associates each would pay $10,000 into a fund that would be the working capital. Those who could not subscribe the full amount in cash would contract to pay the balance over the years from their salaries. The committee estimated $200,000 in cash would be raised. The association would pay 5 percent return on the investment.
* Future associates would each subscribe $10,000 upon entering. Upon the death or resignation of an associate, his subscription would be refunded.
* The association would enter into a contract with the Ochsner Foundation that would be less demanding than the arrangement between the partnership and the foundation. The association's first obligation would be to its employees, not the foundation.
* Association business would be conducted by a medical director and an executive committee composed of three of the original partners and two associates.

Declaring that it neither requested nor anticipated an acknowledgment of its suggestions, the committee included with the memorandum a petition for membership that was signed by twenty-five staff members and by Charles Eshleman, a physician nearing the end of his career who had an employment contract with the clinic. Those who signed, in addition to Eshleman, were Rawley Martin Penick, general surgery; Willoughby E. Kittredge, urology; John C. Weed, obstetrics-gynecology; Edgar H. Little, radiology; Julius Lane Wilson, chest; Theodore L. L. Soniat, psychiatry-neurology; William R. Arrowsmith, hematology; Thomas Findley, medicine; Dean H. Echols, neurosurgery; John Archinard, medicine; William D. Davis, Jr., gastroenterology; Joseph K. Bradford, chest; Merrill O. Hines, colon and rectal surgery; Homer D. Kirgis, neurosurgery; A. J. Ochsner, anesthesiology; Harold Horack, cardiology; Mercer G. Lynch, otolaryngology; Robert C. Lynch, general surgery; Harry D. Morris, orthopedics; Richard Boyer, radiology; Herbery Harms, psychiatry; George Bass Grant, anesthesiology; Idys Mims Gage, general surgery; Lodwick "Locke" Meriwether, endocrinology; and Arthur Seldon Mann, internal medicine.

Blanc Monroe advised rejection of the administrative advisory committee's proposal because he believed it was unnecessary to have additional capital subscribed by associates. In addition, the suggested executive committee was unacceptable to him because two of the founders would be excluded. But he was sympathetic to the thought that clinic salaries should take precedence over foundation claims. He also continued to support changes that would permit more staff participation.

On May 29, the day after the advisory committee submitted its proposal, Guy Caldwell put an effective end to the agitation for reorganizing the clinic into an association. One of the idea's chief attractions was the considerable saving of taxes that an association seemed to offer. Now, Caldwell reported to the partners that it was not legally possible to set up an association with tax-saving features. Furthermore, Caldwell explained, "It seems apparent that many of the staff members who have discussed the association plan as it operates at the Mayo Clinic, the Lovelace Clinic and elsewhere are under the impression that such a plan implies a purely democratic staff organization with Directors elected by the staff and full control of financial policies by the staff. This is not true, and the effect of the association plan as used at the Mayo Clinic and elsewhere is much the same as the modified partnership plan [the plan for an association] now being offered."

Crosscurrents flowed. Although the founders were aware they had reached the age to begin to plan for a transition that would bring senior staff members into the partnership, they did not share their thoughts outside of their own councils. The staff continued to complain that the partners were stern father figures who tended to keep aloof from their employees, professional and lay. "You have built an iron curtain," Merrill Hines told them at a meeting in June. "Part of the staff's dissatisfaction is caused by the fact that the iron curtain has prevented a free discussion of Clinic income and outgo."

Nearly two years after the creation of the administrative advisory committee, the staff won its first direct voting representation in the conduct of clinic affairs. On July 6, 1951, the partners approved a re-organization of the clinic structure, setting up a board of administrators with seven members to have unchallengeable power to make the major decisions. The five founders assumed seats on the board and arranged for the staff to elect two of its senior members to seats. A year later the plan was amended to automatically seat the head of the medical department on the board, leaving only one slot to be filled by election.

The hired doctors had a foot in the door, but the founders had no intention of losing control. They made sure that five votes were required for any board action. Nevertheless, the new plan gave the staff much more input into day-by-day operations. The table of organization included a staff executive committee composed of nine staff members selected by the board of administrators. This committee was charged with carrying out the policies set by the board and was given broad powers—including hiring and firing—although it could be overridden by the administrators. The staff executive committee was regarded as the successor to the administrative advisory committee, but with more clout.

The name *administrative advisory committee* was now conferred on a panel made up of foundation trustees Blanc Monroe and Theodore Brent and one of the two staff doctors on the board of administrators. It was an outgrowth of the executive committee dominated by laymen to which the partners had surrendered much of the fiscal responsibility of the clinic during the spring of 1951. Although the committee was advisory in name, it was more influential than the title would suggest. Rules made it mandatory for the board of administrators to seek the advisory committee's advice and recommendations on important decisions. Monroe and, to a somewhat smaller extent, Brent participated in foundation matters as trustees. As members of the administrative advisory committee, they could also affect clinic affairs. And of course, Brent was a director of the Hibernia National Bank, to which the clinic was indebted.

Here were the five founders having outside laymen looking over one shoulder, and hired employees over the other. Their tolerance of such an arrangement proved their complete dedication to the success of the enterprise they had created.

Two months later, the founders made yet another change aimed at improving staff morale. They replaced the business manager. When Junius Underwood was hired as the first lay employee of the clinic, Caldwell told him that his title "would not be 'M.D.,' but 'S.B.'" Finally, he was asked to leave because the founders felt he had interpreted Caldwell's remark too literally.

Underwood, an architect who had previously operated a collection agency for physicians, was taken on as business manager in 1941 during the organization period. First, he visited the major clinics to study their administrative procedures. Another of his early assignments was to negotiate with tenants of the building at 3503 Prytania. Most had to move in order to ensure ample office space for the opening of the clinic on the day after New Year's, 1942.

Underwood had a voice in the founders' councils, and he established the early business practices of the clinic. He joined Dean H. Echols in advocating the chartering of a nonprofit foundation, and was named to the additional job of manager of the Alton Ochsner Medical Foundation at the first meeting on January 17, 1944. Apparently his problems began to accumulate in 1945 when, he later admitted, "I was guilty of not handling my duties well. . . . Dr. Caldwell very kindly told me so in dutch uncle fashion—for which I am eternally grateful." Two years later the partners voted him a token raise in salary, and Caldwell said they felt the manager was doing a good job. In the financial crisis of 1950–1951, however, Underwood was blamed, rightly or wrongly, for failing to make the partners aware of the seriousness of the situation.

But the ax fell because of his relationships with lay employees. When the partners instructed him to pare expenses, he chose to freeze salaries and reduce sick benefits. The professional staff was already near revolt because of low pay, and now the morale of nurses, receptionists, secretaries, and record clerks plummeted. Caldwell held confidential conferences with a dozen of the senior employees and filed a report to the other founders. He told of complaints that Underwood was an "absolute dictator," who was "abrupt, inconsiderate and harsh." Often, he would wait near the front of the clinic in the morning to catch latecomers as they entered. Employees had devised a system to avoid confronting Underwood and receiving a dressing down. Whenever the manager took his station near the door, somebody would display a towel at a second-floor window. Forewarned, tardy employees would duck around the building and enter from the rear. The unhappy situation was compounded by the reduction in pay and benefits. Caldwell recommended that the business manager be replaced.

Underwood sought support from the one man who might have saved his job, Blanc Monroe. The manager wrote for the partners this account of a meeting with the attorney-trustee.

> Before I had a chance to say anything, Mr. Monroe had this to say: "Junius, I want you to know that until Dr. Caldwell informed me of this action I knew nothing of it. My only reply to him was to question if he had a replacement as good as Junius. He said he had no one in mind. I cautioned him to go slowly because Junius Underwood has done a splendid job." Then I was able to ask him if he and Mr. Brent were dissatisfied. He said he could speak for himself with certainty, and, so far as he knew, for Mr. Brent, "that to the contrary he was highly satisfied with me and was keenly disappointed with the doctors' decision."
>
> I reminded him that he may have been unhappy during the recent meetings concerning the Clinic's financial crisis. He replied that, "Junius, you and George Conroy know me well enough to know that I always fume and fuss over orthodox reports—that I am peculiar about my figures—and I always send you back and back again until you produce what I want in my own unorthodox way. It is possible that one of the doctors may have interpreted this as 'dissatisfaction' but actually I am completely satisfied and think that you co-operated splendidly in a most difficult and trying problem that took at least five days of my time."

Nevertheless, in August, 1951, Caldwell told Underwood, "I am afraid we have come to a parting of the ways." On September 17, in a memorandum to the staff, Caldwell announced that Underwood had resigned. He said Underwood had been with the clinic since it began and had "contributed much toward its development and success." Indeed, the circumstances of his departure should not obscure the fact that Underwood is due part of the credit for the promising beginning of the Ochsner Institutions.

Fund Raising Succeeds

In 1951, while the founders and the staff worked out a way to continue the Ochsner Institutions, Raymond T. Rich and Associates changed its fund-raising tactics. Rich culled a list of prospective donors throughout the South from the roster of former Ochsner patients. Out of 100,000 patients from the states of Louisiana, Texas, Arkansas, Mississippi, Alabama, Florida, and Georgia, 787 appeared to rate as likely donors. Rich arranged for Ochsner Clinic doctors to visit many of these former patients to make personal appeals for funds. After all, in its first decade, the Ochsner center had established a reputation among southerners and was getting a sizable share of its practice from word-of-mouth referrals by patients. And patients responded to the appeals. From another list of 412 prospects, drawn up by the public relations office, 138 made contributions totaling $108,105.

Staff members fanned out on hurried visits to prospective donors in south-central and southeastern states, at the same time continuing to cover their full schedule of patient appointments at the clinic. Sometimes it was a weary, sleepy-eyed physician or surgeon who showed up at his office after a long automobile drive the night before. Once, on a foray into the Florida Panhandle, Merrill Hines was speeding home at midnight when the engine of his old-model car became overheated from a radiator leak. Pulling to the side of the road, Hines spotted a bridge a hundred yards ahead. He dipped water from the stream with the only container he had—his Rex Harrison–style hat—and drove slowly to the nearest service station. He pounded on the door until he roused the proprietor, who responded to the doctor's plea that he had sick people to see in New Orleans as soon as he could get there. A leaky water hose was replaced, and Hines made it to the clinic on time.

Part of the medical clan persisted in considering the Ochsner group a Judas. The notion that once a physician's patient entered an Ochsner building, he was lost forever, still prevailed, although the clinic tried from the beginning to guard against any appearance of patient-stealing. Strict rules required that a referring doctor be sent full and prompt reports on his patient. Clinic members took part in the activities of specialty associations and the national, state, and local medical societies. Ochsner was in no way a medical maverick. Yet if the clinic and foundation had depended principally on outside referrals for their patients, they wouldn't have needed the present campus. Nowadays, hundreds of practitioners who received fellowship training at Ochsner are scattered throughout the country; they provide the facility with a cadre of friends that was not nearly as large in 1951.

But Alton Ochsner's dependable Presbyterian luck stayed with him. Congress completed action on the Hill-Burton Act, enabling the foundation to turn to the state of Louisiana for an allocation of federal funds. And when the campaign for donations showed signs of flagging, Theodore Brent came forward with a $400,000 gift that restored the momentum. On August 3, 1951, William H. Helis, Jr., announced that he would equip the new hospital laboratories as a memorial to his father. The basic twenty-one-acre tract of the present campus, now with the address 1514–1516 Jefferson Highway, was purchased on December 20, 1951, from the Illinois Central Railroad at a cost of $6,000 per acre. It was known as the Riding Academy site, for ponies were stabled on the grounds, and a ring provided a training track for neophyte equestrians.

The foundation trustees prepared to clear the final financial hurdle by obtaining a $1 million mortgage loan. They had begun negotiations with the Massachusetts Mutual Life Insurance Company when Howell Crosby suggested that they approach Crawford H. Ellis, president of the Pan-American Life Insurance Company of New Orleans. Pan-American granted a loan under favorable terms, and in early 1951 Ellerbe and Company of St. Paul, Minnesota, architectural specialists in medical buildings, was engaged to prepare plans for the hospital. On May 27, 1952, the trustees completed arrangements with the contractors, Farnsworth and Chambers, for construction of the building. The first piling was driven on July 2, 1952.

On September 21, 1953, with the first building on the new campus nearing completion, the trustees of the Alton Ochsner Medical Foundation changed the name of the hospital to the Ochsner Foundation

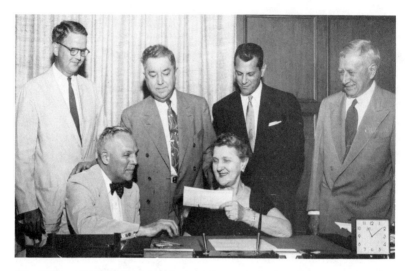

Mrs. William G. Helis presents a check to Alton Ochsner for $250,000 payable to the Alton Ochsner Medical Foundation. Seated behind them, *left to right*: Richard Freeman; Dr. Robert Bernhard, trustee of the Helis Foundation; William G. Helis, Jr., trustee of the Helis Foundation; and J. Blanc Monroe

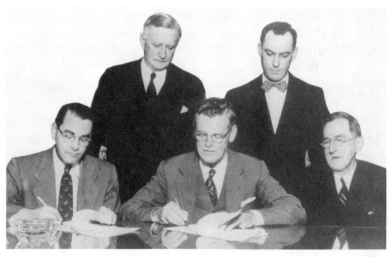

Executing the act of sale of the Riding Academy site. *Left to right*: Harry V. Souchon, agent and attorney for the Illinois Central Railroad; J. Blanc Monroe; Guy A. Caldwell; Bat P. Sullivan, attorney and notary public; and Theodore Brent.

Hospital. The name better identified the facility with the clinic. It also announced the proud tradition that the hospital would uphold.

As the building progressed, a boom began to transform the East Bank of Jefferson Parish from a sleepy suburb into one of the busiest, most populous, most affluent communities in the South. Ochsner had chosen its site wisely. Some of the prospects that had seemed ideal in 1950 are now in decaying neighborhoods or would be too cramped to accommodate today's demands. For nearly two decades New Orleans expanded to the west, and the Riding Academy site put the new hospital in the path of this growth. The scene was set not merely for survival but for success.

CHAPTER SEVEN

The Ownership Is Shared

By 1955 the foundation was settled in a new hospital, and the staff crises of the 1949–1952 era lay behind the clinic. The founders were getting old: Guy Caldwell would turn sixty-five on January 24, 1956, and the others were either in or approaching their sixties. The time had come for decisions.

Off on a vacation trip, Caldwell sat down in Los Angeles and wrote a letter to administrator Edgar J. Saux. At the heart of the problem lay two fundamental questions that had to be settled in 1956: how and to what extent the staff should participate in sharing future clinic policy and earnings and how the present partnership could be terminated and the partners paid off without loading the new organization with a debilitating debt.

> The future security and stability of the clinic (and foundation) depend upon having full, whole-hearted interest and cooperation of the staff and key personnel. (By staff, I mean those with 5+ years of service.) This I believe can only be realized by *real* participation, both in policy making and profit sharing. This would require a *very* large partnership with a very complicated formula for voting and sharing. It cannot be visualized and made acceptable *if* full control is to be retained by a small minority of older members. With a tight, small controlling group we will never be able to recruit the top-flight men required to do the kind of work we wish to have done. An association is the *only* real answer to this problem. . . . I know that JBM [Monroe] will never agree to this. . . . There might be little or no difference in the money paid & the terms of payment, but I think it would make a great difference in the thinking and attitude of the

entire staff who must share the responsibility for paying off the debt and at the same time to try to provide for better staff income and future expansion. If *all* the staff *elects* the board that decides these matters, they will be much more willing to accept the restrictions than if control is left in the hands of a *few* who by pull or purchase get themselves made senior partners. . . . The staff thinking and attitude is what really controls our services to patients and our income & unless the staff is satisfied & have a feeling of real participation, the future of the Clinic is not secure nor sound.

Every time the founding partners had tried to bring clinic and foundation under a single association for which all of the doctors would work on salary, Monroe had blocked the change. Now, from a distance of two thousand miles, Caldwell was defiant. When he got home, his resolve had not melted, and he found the other partners willing to join him in a showdown. On April 28, 1955, all five signed a letter to Monroe.

You have indicated that you are ready, as soon as your time permits, to advise with the five partners as to the best plan for terminating the present partnership and providing for a future succession and defining its relations to the Foundation. We shall be glad to have this opportunity and, as always, will be grateful for your advice. In approaching this discussion, however, we wish to have you understand clearly what we and our staff doctors consider to be our proper objectives and responsibilities. We believe that these differ somewhat from the objectives which you have in mind and unless we first agree that certain goals are right and proper we are likely to talk at cross purposes in discussing ways and means to achieve them.

When we established the Clinic we did so because we were convinced that a carefully selected group of specialists working together could provide the best medical care possible for patients at the most reasonable costs. "Maximum medical care at minimal costs to the patient" was to be our slogan. After thirteen years of experience we are still convinced that group practice is the best way to achieve this end but we believe that we are failing to furnish the best medical care at the least possible cost and now that we are in a position to do so, we wish to alter our course to head more directly towards our original goal.

Deviation from the course originally set was caused by circumstances beyond our control and we believe that the progress that has been made in spite of contrary winds and unforeseen difficulties is in large part due to your wise guidance and help. But now that the worst of the storm has passed we wish to correct our course and proceed in the direction originally planned.

The epistle—the style of which makes Caldwell's authorship obvious—noted that the founders had at the start no intention of operating a hospital but were finally forced by circumstances to open Splinter Village. For seven years the old army hospital was subsidized by the clinic. The total out-of-pocket cost to the clinic for keeping the Foundation Hospital in business until the new hospital could be built was $947,000. Equipment valued at $160,000 was salvaged for the present hospital, and the buildings of Splinter Village were sold for $46,000. Thus the net cost to the clinic was $741,000, averaging $106,000 per year. This money, the letter continued,

> was realized from our Clinic patients as increased charges, and from our staff and personnel by suppressing their salaries, and by withholding needed new equipment and limiting expansion of our facilities. Therefore all rejoice in the fact that the new hospital has been donated to us by the public and ardently hope that it can be operated by the Board of Governors with no deficits to be met by Clinic. It is a matter of grave concern to the entire staff that Clinic patients, the majority of whom are *not* referred to the hospital for care, must be taxed to help maintain a hospital for those who do require hospitalization. This definitely defeats our purpose to provide the best care at the lowest possible cost. The staff reasons that we should be in the same position as are other specialists and groups in New Orleans and throughout the country, viz., that hospital facilities built by the public are available to them without cost to themselves or to their non-hospital patients. When such community and church hospitals operate with a deficit they do not ask their staff members to help meet it from their earnings, and if there be a loan that requires amortization the Trustees do not undertake to assess the staff and their office patients to make the payments.
>
> Therefore we, the partners, and our staff would like the Trustees of the Foundation and the Board of Governors to operate Foundation Hospital as far as possible without obligating the Clinic for funds. Since the funds for building the hospital have been donated by the public and since it is rapidly becoming recognized as a community enterprise, we hope that the citizens of this area can be educated to support it as they do other

hospitals—not expecting the Clinic to absorb its losses. We accept the fact that we are now obligated by written agreement to meet the deficits but we wish to steer in the direction of becoming free of this obligation as soon as possible in order that the Clinic may be fairer to its patients in making its charges and that Clinic's income may be available to pay better salaries to its personnel and staff and to provide better facilities as needed.

The founders called for a reappraisal of the educational and research activities of the foundation and the extent to which the clinic, in all fairness, should be expected to support them.

When we established the Foundation in 1944 by donating our equities in the buildings, grounds and equipment and then made a rental agreement, we did so in the belief that the modest income thus provided for the Foundation would suffice to support a few fellowships, one or two small laboratories for research, and hospital expenses for a few patients having treatment problems of special interest. This it did very well during the early years, but when Foundation acquired the hospital it also rapidly expanded its Educational program and its research, all of which has grown far beyond the ability of the Clinic to support from reasonable rentals and donations. Fortunately, some support has been realized from donations from individuals and by special grants from various sources, but in spite of these, Foundation's programs other than its hospital, are far more expensive than Clinic can afford to support by fair rentals and reasonable donations. Unless we can succeed in obtaining public support for much of the Foundation's work we should seriously consider curtailing them. Therefore, before the budget for another fiscal year is approved and before new lease contracts between Foundation and Clinic are made, we, the partners and our staff request that charges to Clinic be made *minimal* and that the Foundation budget for the coming year be curtailed in proportion if necessary.

Finally, the partners turned to the matter of reorganizing the clinic.

For many good reasons we wish to terminate the present partnership and establish a new administration capable of assuming the obligations of the present group and also capable of purchasing the accounts receivable and paying for them gradually over a period of years. This step we believe to be absolutely essential for future security of the Clinic. We are under obligations to our staff members, many of whom have shared in the struggle to place Clinic and Foundation on a firm financial basis, to give them an opportunity to take part in the administration and to share in the profits. Since the five partners are nearing retirement age we owe it no less to our creditors and the public to provide a gradual transfer of control and responsibility to our younger associates. We are convinced that this step should be taken before any projects [*sic*] such as the construction of a new clinic building is undertaken. We therefore urge that this be done along with the other foregoing steps.

Five days after the letter was written, it fell to Caldwell's lot to face Monroe without the supportive presence of the other partners. The two were joined in a meeting by trustee Richard Freeman, accountant George E. Conroy, and administrator Edgar Saux. Monroe reminded Caldwell that the clinic had obligated itself to the government, the Pan-American Life Insurance Company, and those who had contributed funds for the new hospital when it agreed to absorb any operating deficits. Any change in the clinic organization therefore would have to be made with the consent of these interested parties. Freeman and Conroy agreed with Monroe that a partnership would be better understood and accepted than any other arrangement. Monroe also questioned whether an association would offer any tax advantages and warned against asking the Internal Revenue Service for a change in tax status. He still believed that such a move would stir hostile elements in the medical profession to seek legislation that would be disadvantageous to Ochsner. Nevertheless, Monroe and the others agreed that the drain on the clinic should be reduced. The founders and early staff members had made sacrifices to establish and maintain a center that became a national health resource. Now, support for the training and research activities must come as well from the public that was benefiting.

By the end of May, 1955, planning for the expansion of the partnership was in progress. For thirteen years the founders had not benefited financially from their burgeoning brainchild beyond their equal draws, or salaries, which had always been moderate in the scale of incomes among New Orleans surgeons and physicians. They could have grown rich from a commercial business doing the same dollar volume or at least well-to-do had the clinic not been burdened by the foundation.

The founders could look forward with pleasure to their long overdue payday, but first a complicated arrangement had to be worked out.

The partners had donated all of the clinic's property to the foundation; they paid rent on buildings, furniture, and equipment. The clinic's sole asset was the accounts receivable. These could be converted into cash, but they also represented the only operating funds. The staff members who would come into the expanded partnership were all salaried men, hardly one of them with enough savings to pay cash for a share. Somehow, the founders would have to be reimbursed for a part of their interests, the staff members would have to acquire their shares mostly on credit, and the clinic would have to retain enough working capital to pay salaries and expenses without plunging into oppressive debt.

In addition, the founders, whose own efforts had created a major medical center, understandably felt proprietorship for the institutions that were the fruits of their lives' work. It was not easy to give up even a part of their ownership. Like all successful men, they enjoyed the thought of having something valuable to pass along to their heirs. Three of Alton Ochsner's sons had chosen medical careers. Francis LeJeune's son and namesake was an otolaryngologist, and his son-in-law, George T. Schneider, was an obstetrician-gynecologist. Guy Caldwell, Edgar Burns, and Curtis Tyrone had no physician sons, but Tyrone had a fatherly interest in his long-time associate and protégé, John C. Weed, who was already on the ob-gyn staff. It was natural enough for the founders to hope these young physicians, to whom they were so close, would succeed them in the enterprise that had been central in their own lives.

Discussions lasted for months before a plan could be worked out that the founders could unanimously support. As usual five strong individualists had to reach a consensus. Something of how the founders worked together through their years of active service at Ochsner can be glimpsed in one of Guy Caldwell's many memoranda—this one written during the planning for the expanded partnership.

Curtis Tyrone had proposed a requirement that all partners spend an equal amount of time in the clinic. Additionally, he wanted all partners to agree to turn over to the clinic any income they earned for professional services outside the clinic. The other four discussed the suggestions among themselves and unanimously agreed that they were undesirable. Edgar Burns was designated to report the reaction to Tyrone. He did so, then suggested that Alton Ochsner and Caldwell confer with Tyrone about the matter. The three met on a Sunday morning, and Tyrone got some complaints off his chest. He said he regretted that Burns and Francis LeJeune were not present because he and they represented a majority of the partners and their requests should be put into effect. Caldwell's handwritten memorandum to the absent founders took up Tyrone's points, one by one.

> C. T. is available in Clinic most days from 9–5; sees 350–400 patients per month. Of these he believes 25% are referred to other departments. This is *hard* work and represents far more time spent in Clinic than other partners give & undoubtedly contributes considerably to Clinic income outside his own department. C. T. finds himself acting as an appointment desk for referral of patients and believes that he does not get proper recognition & remuneration for this work. Because he works longer hours in Clinic, is away from home much less than the other partners & consequently personally sees more patients than the others & refers many patients to other departments or for clinic checks & the income thus derived is not reflected in the department of gynecology, & because he has no income from any other source outside the Clinic, he believes his salary should be increased.
>
> C. T. further believes that had he continued in private practice instead of joining Clinic partnership, he would have realized a much larger income. He is the youngest member of the group and believes that it would be to his personal advantage to now withdraw & resume private practice. Therefore, if he is to continue as a partner under the new agreement, he wishes the others to consider one of two alternatives.
>
> a. Other partners to stay at home & give as many hours to Clinic work as he does, or
>
> b. Increased income to C. T. as compensation for the added time he spends in Clinic.

Caldwell noted that statistics bore out Tyrone's contention that he saw more patients than any of the others and that his referrals of seventy-five to a hundred patients a month to other departments exceed those of the others.

Under our present agreement, all partners contributed equally to the capital investment and all were to participate equally in the profits. It then was recognized that the practice brought into Clinic by each of the five differed greatly, that Al Ochsner received a full time salary from Tulane and devoted more time to his teaching than any other member. However, it was generally accepted that he should retain his teaching position and receive the salary from the school in addition to an equal share of the Clinic earnings. The principle was also accepted that there would probably always be considerable difference in the earnings of the various partners in their respective departments and that the amount of teaching & absences from Clinic to attend meetings etc. would vary greatly. Nevertheless, we agreed that the prestige & drawing power of the Clinic as a whole would be greatly enhanced by teaching at Tulane and by participating prominently in the national and regional medical meetings, therefore no agreement was made to require partners to spend an equal amount of time in Clinic and no consideration has been given to distributing profits in proportion to the earnings of various departments.

Curtis Tyrone has requested reconsideration of this part of the agreement on at least two other occasions & has emphasized the fact that because he spends more time in Clinic than others, that he should receive a greater income. Our reply has been that our agreement has not required him to do this, that he has been at liberty to attend meetings or have more time away from Clinic if he desired, but we did not agree that the contributions of the other partners towards increasing the drawing power & prestige of Clinic by these outside activities were less than his. The same decision was made again when the four partners read and considered Curtis' letter on this point, but he is still not satisfied.

The always conciliatory Caldwell said adjustments would soon have to be made because of partial or complete retirement of some partners, and perhaps Tyrone should receive as much as $6,000 a year in additional income if he continued to spend more time in the clinic than the others did.

To Tyrone's complaint that he needed an experienced nurse and a junior staff man to help with his patients, Caldwell said Tyrone had been advised that if he could find a nurse who would satisfy him, she would be hired. Caldwell suggested that Tyrone find a suitable junior man and request that the board of administrators add him to the staff. The memorandum continued:

Curtis personally has had repeated difficulty in obtaining direct appointments for his patients referred to surgery & also thru the appointment desk. This he attributes in part to Al Ochsner's frequent absences from the school that make it necessary for some staff men to cancel their hours in Clinic in order to cover Al's work at School. Al Ochsner agrees that this should not happen.

Curtis also criticizes surgery for assigning operations to junior staff men that should be assigned to the more experienced men. Dr. Ochsner believes that his junior men are fully capable of doing every case assigned. Comment,—Al Ochsner is probably correct as to the ability of his junior staff members to perform the operations assigned to them, and this practice would be acceptable for a charity service—However, the important question with the private patient is whether or not he (the patient & the family) are satisfied to be referred. . . .

C. T. criticizes the medical department for having some staff men with poor personalities, (unable to sell themselves to their patients) and believes that the women doctors should probably see only women. He also believes there should be a mechanism whereby V.I.P. patients should be carefully referred to suitable senior members of various departments.

Comment: The desirability & need of some stronger, more experienced staff members in the medical department has been generally recognized for a long time & undoubtedly we have added weaker members from our own fellowship group thru expediency rather than good judgment & largely because the needs were urgent and the salaries we could afford to offer are low. Now that they are a part of the staff we are faced with the problem of dismissing them without having obvious reasons & obtaining suitable replacements at salaries proportionate to those of the older staff men in the departments. To improve this situation will require (1) Careful review of the entire budget and salary scale for all staff members (2) Search for suitable replacements at the salary that can be offered (3) Approach to problems of dismissing those considered to be incompetent. If most of us agree that these steps should be taken, we should present the need at a meeting of the Bd of Administrators & discuss with Dr. [William R.] Arrowsmith & with his consent, review and increase the budget for his department. He, together with the personnel committee, should then consider those to be replaced & proceed.

Limitation of the assignment of patients to the women doctors in medicine should also be discussed with the Bd of Adm & Dr. Arrowsmith before any directives are given to the section heads and the appointment desk. When Dr. Margaret Shelton was given a staff appointment, the entire question was discussed at a meeting of our board, and with Drs. Arrow-smith and [Lodwick S.] Meriwether and all agreed to her appointment altho I consented with great reluctance and apprehension. However, so long as we have women assigned to the staff in internal medicine, I think it will not be practical to restrict them to seeing only female patients.

Establishment of a mechanism for referral of V.I.P. patients to senior members of the various departments is desirable in a limited number of cases. The need has been recently discussed, but no workable solution has been found. It would require an experienced physician or very su-perior nurse to give full time to the direction of such cases & that this person be given authority to alter routine appointments & "force" ap-pointments in many instances. Even when managed with all possible di-plomacy, it would create friction & resentment in many instances and would not always satisfy the V.I.P. It could and probably would lead to abuse & if abused, would certainly lead to confusion and turmoil. Every member of our staff should, ideally, be good enough to handle any V.I.P.

The financial crisis caused by a slump in patient visits and the de-mands of the foundation on the clinic for support was still a problem when Caldwell wrote his memorandum. More recently, the clinic has paid salaries in the upper ranges of the going rate and hired only doc-tors whose competence makes them able to pass specialty board ex-amination. The number of women on the staff corresponds to the pro-portion in medical practice who qualify as specialists. Any patient, including very important persons, may request the services of any staff doctor, but the clinic's policy now is that any physician or surgeon on the staff is capable of treating any patient who falls within his spe-cialty area.

Tyrone complained that partners had no opportunity to present their viewpoint or get a proper hearing at meetings of the trustees. "I do not understand why this criticism is directed to me since I do not preside at the meetings," Caldwell wrote.

If you believe that thru preliminary conferences for procurement of data, i.e. estimates, bids & other pertinent information matters of policy are "cut and dried" & railroaded thru at formal meetings you are wrong. Even if I wished to do so, J.B.M. [Blanc Monroe] & Dick F. [Richard Freeman] would never permit such steps. In order to conserve time of partners & J.B.M., I *do* try to have all essential data obtained & preliminary steps taken, so that a given problem is ready for final discussion and decision by the Full Board. Once a decision on policy is given, the details of putting it into effect are carried on as far as possible without further discussion. You are aware that in all matters of financial policy of the Foundation or between Clinic and Foundation J.B.M. confers with R.F. & they have made their own decisions prior to any meeting of the full Board. Sometimes I am in agreement with them, other times I am not, and I do not always know their combined thinking prior to our meetings. J.B.M. uses his full powers of persuasion & argument to get approval for what he considers right and best. If we permit him to impose his will and judgment upon us at the open meetings when decisions are reached it is our own fault.

Certainly each of you know [*sic*] that more often than not I have joined you in opposing many of his policies and have sought to improve Clinic's relation to Foundation. Actually, only thru repeated strong protests which I have voiced and written have we succeeded in

1. Getting partners released from guarantee of mortgage
2. Getting bed credits abolished
3. Getting hospital deficits reduced
4. Getting part of cost of fellows transferred to hospital
5. Cutting down or withholding donations to Foundation until Cl. [clinic] debts are paid
6. Providing insurance & fair salaries in order to keep our staff intact.

These steps together with good management by Ed Saux have more than doubled the value of our respective interests in accounts receivable & every step has been taken in spite of J.B.M.'s opposition.

If these gloomy passages read like the requiem for an enterprise that was about to be ripped asunder by internal conflict, do not be misled. Alton Ochsner used to explain that the partners went 'round and 'round behind closed doors, and always emerged to present a united front. Curtis Tyrone bowed to the decision of the others not to give him extra pay and contiued to work as hard as always. Patients came in ever-increasing numbers, requiring development of the Jefferson Highway campus. The staff more than doubled in size. The troubles that were so vexing at the time were only growing pains, long since cured.

A plan was at long last worked out for the new partnership. The agreement was scheduled to take effect at the beginning of the fiscal year, May 1, 1956. A hitch developed in the granting of approval by the Internal Revenue Service, however, and so the new partnership came into being on May 1, 1957. Actually, final IRS authorization came on July 8, 1957.

Thirty-two doctors who had served the clinic for five years or longer became partners, each acquiring a ¹⁄₆₄th interest. The five original partners each retained a ¹⁄₁₀th share, since the ownership was divided on the basis of half for the founders and half for the new men. The new partners each put up $1,000 in cash and signed a three-year promissory note for $2,729.10 in payment for his share. (By 1982, when the number of partners had increased to 109, out of a total professional staff of 184, the value of a partnership had increased to $169,614.) All of the accounts receivable by the clinic on April 30, 1957, were credited to the original five. The estimated cash value of the accounts was $487,005.42, and the total buy-in cost to the new partners was $119,331.20. Thus the price for one-half of the clinic was a total of $606,336.62. This provided something like $121,267.32 for each of the founders. The exact total would vary a little, depending on the actual collections of the accounts receivable and the interest on the new partners' notes.

Upon reaching retirement age, each of the founders was to be paid his remaining one-tenth share in the clinic's assets. Dr. Tyrone received $162,701.60, for instance, and the others took home comparable amounts. The 1957 partnership agreement also provided for each founder, while he worked, to receive an annual income of $24,750, on which the income tax would be paid by the clinic. In fact, the highest pay ever given to a founder was $42,500 a year, tax free. These sums looked larger in the years before inflation moved into double digit ground, but it was apparent even then that starting a New Orleans clinic was no road to riches.

The first staff members who bought into the new partnership were John J. Archinard, William R. Arrowsmith, John Butler Blalock, Robert Birchall, Joseph K. Bradford, Buell C. Buchtel, Walter S. Culpepper, William D. Davis, Jr., Paul T. DeCamp, Thomas L. Duncan, Dean H. Echols, George B. Grant, Patrick H. Hanley, Merrill O. Hines, Harold M. Horack, Homer D. Kirgis, Willoughby E. Kittredge, Francis X. LeTard, Miles L. Lewis, Jr., Edgar H. Little, William Locke, Mercer G. Lynch, Robert C. Lynch, A. Seldon Mann, Harry D. Morris, Paul J.

Murison, Rawley M. Penick, George T. Schneider, C. Harrison Snyder, Theodore L. L. Soniat, John C. Weed, and Thomas E. Weiss. The partnership was also open to future members. The agreement provided that when a doctor completed five years on the staff, his name would be submitted to the partnership. If three-fourths of the members voted affirmatively, he would be allowed to buy a pro rata interest in the clinic's assets.

There were now thirty-seven partners instead of five, but the founders made no pretense of yielding control immediately. A board of management was created and given the same broad powers that the board of administrators had always wielded. All five of the original partners were placed on the seven-man board. Two of the new partners—William R. Arrowsmith and Rawley M. Penick—were elected by their fellows to continue in the board seats they already occupied.

Frank Lahey, that outspoken advocate of autocratic control, would have applauded the board of management regulations Monroe had written into the partnership agreement. Members were given ten-year terms, and the board was set up to be almost self-perpetuating. In the event of a vacancy, the remaining members would nominate a successor. The nominee would be seated unless rejected by two-thirds of the partners. Not until 1971 were the provisions changed to provide for direct election of board members.

Monroe also saw to it that board action required five favorable votes. The founders' long experience at thrashing out their differences privately and always presenting a united front in public gave them a sharp advantage in board debates. Obviously, they would still have decisive influence in clinic affairs, even if the new partners dissented. But the arrangement was palatable to the staff because it would be only temporary. The agreement made it mandatory for every board member to step down at the age of seventy. This meant that only Curtis Tyrone was eligible to serve out a full ten-year term. The others would have to yield their places earlier.

The first to go was Caldwell, who was succeeded on April 30, 1960, by Merrill Hines. The founders were left with a four-to-three majority until August 10, 1964, when LeJeune gave up his seat. After that, the three remaining founders theoretically could block a board action by staying together and denying the required fifth vote, although in prac-

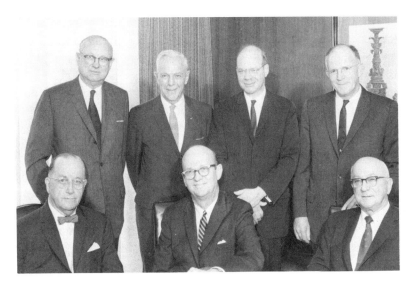

Founders and successors. *Back row*: Curtis Tyrone, Alton Ochsner, William Davis, and William Arrowsmith; *front row*: Edgar Burns, Merrill Hines, and Francis LeJeune

tice the senior men were influential and there was no face-off between old and new partners. Upon the retirement of Burns on April 30, 1966, the new partners acquired their fifth member, in effect taking the affairs of the clinic from the hands of the old guard. Ochsner waited only until his seventieth birthday on May 4, five days after Burns's withdrawal, before relinquishing his own board membership, and Tyrone retired on April 30, 1968. Although after retirement they had no votes, the founders were allowed to continue attending board of management meetings and taking part in the discussions.

During the early years of the clinic, there had been anxiety over the financial problems that would result from the death of a partner and the necessity of turning over his share of the assets to his estate. Insurance policies were carried to ease the burden. As it turned out, the worries were unnecessary. The five doctors all lived long enough to have their claims against the clinic satisfied, and indeed, all proved remarkably long-lived. Only Burns, who died at seventy-eight, failed to survive into his eighties, and Caldwell was nearing ninety-one when he succumbed to the infirmities of old age.

The partnership agreement had allowed the founders another decade of deep involvement in the affairs of the Ochsner Institutions. More important, it had permitted a smooth transition as age forced the founders into retirement and the second-generation partners gradually took over management. But this second generation was composed of men not much younger than the founders, and so its tenure in power was briefer than that of the founders.

Thirteen years after the formation of the new partnership, the question of whether the clinic should become a professional corporation or merge into the foundation came up for renewed debate. On April 21, 1970, the partners heard a discussion of the alternatives. They were told they could transfer their shares of the partnership assets into stock in a professional corporation, which now would present none of the legal problems Blanc Monroe had once feared. But the change would result in income bunching in which each partner would have to pay, in one calendar year, the income tax on twenty months of earnings. If the partnership were liquidated and the doctors became employees of the foundation, they would have to yield their shares of the clinic's assets. Those at the meeting voted unanimously to retain the partnership plan that Monroe had devised nearly thirty years earlier.

Records of the Louisiana secretary of state show that in 1969 the Ochsner Clinic obtained a charter that would allow it to practice as a professional corporation. The structure was set up only as a shell to facilitate reorganization in the event the partnership was ever abolished.

In choosing to retain the partnership, the clinic remained among a minority of the nearly eleven thousand group practices in America. Most of them by far (70.6 percent) are professional corporations. Only 16.7 percent are Ochsner-type partnerships. The others have various legal setups; a few are even sole proprietorships of individual doctors.

For three years after the last of the founders gave up his vote on the board of management, second-generation staff members, those who came into the partnership in 1957, remained in control of clinic affairs. They were able to maintain their control because they could, in effect, name their successors. Never was a two-thirds majority of partners mustered against a board nominee, and so the dynastic succession was left undisturbed.

Then, on May 1, 1971, a new partnership agreement turned the clinic into what might be described as a limited democracy and gave the younger staff a louder voice. The autocratic leadership had carried the group through the formative years. Now, it was recognized, fresh thinking was needed to steer the clinic through the changing tides of modern medicine.

Among the seventy-two partners who signed the new agreement that became effective on May 1, 1971, were second-generation partners Arrowsmith, Blalock, Birchall, Bradford, Culpepper, Davis, De-Camp, Duncan, Dunn, Hanley, Hines, Horack, Kirgis, Kittredge, Le-Tard, Little, Locke, Robert Lynch, Mann, Morris, Murison, Schneider, Snyder, Soniat, Weed, and Weiss. Signers whose signatures had not been affixed to the 1957 document were Robert E. Barron, Hugh Batson, Ralph B. Bergeron, William Brannan, Mario Calonje, Ana Carrera, Guillermo Carrera, Herbert Christianson, William P. Coleman, R. Harold Cox, Fernand Dastugue, Jr., William A. Ferrante, Julio E. Figueroa, George Fruthaler, William Geary, Hurst B. Hatch, John P. Holland, Alan McK. Holtzman, Charles M. Kantrow, Arvil M. Kirk, Richard K. Lange, George Leonard, Francis E. LeJeune, Jr., Gordon McFarland, Duncan McKee, William M. P. McKinnon, Joseph F. Mabey, William T. Mitchell, Charles B. Moore, John Ochsner, Mims Ochsner, Seymour Ochsner, George A. Pankey, George H. Porter III, Virginia Porter, James H. Quinn, C. Thorpe Ray, Frank A. Riddick, Jr., Don Samples, Robert Schimek, Stanton E. Shuler, Andrew H. Thalheim, Jr., Roger H. Tutton, Samuel G. Welborn, and Philip C. Young. Of these, Riddick and Porter, who helped draft the agreement, would emerge as the leaders of the third generation. Porter would subsequently become president of the foundation, and in 1975 Riddick would succeed Merrill Hines as medical director. As such, he would be endowed with the powers that the 1971 pact had formally deeded to the director, powers that Guy Caldwell and Hines had secured over the years. Once elected by the partners, the medical director, by far the most important figure in the clinic administration, now automatically becomes chairman of the board of management.

The other six members of the board of management are elected for seven-year terms by a somewhat complicated process intended to assure some continuity in clinic policies while giving all segments of the partnership representation. When there is to be a vacancy on the board, the first step is for all partners to vote for a successor. The existing nominating commiteee then certifies the names of the four, five, or six partners who received the most votes. At the time of the first ballot the partners also vote for three members of a new nominating committee. One committeeman is elected from each of three categories: doctors who have been partners for more than twenty years, those who have been partners for from ten to twenty years, and those who have been partners for less than ten years. Two other members of the five-man committee are named by the board of management.

The new nominating committee selects two names from among those of the four, five, or six partners who received the most ballots in the original election. The two are not necessarily the top vote-getters, the count being a secret. In another election the partners choose between the two nominees.

Few limitations are placed on the actions of the board of management, four members of which can even unseat the medical director. A member whose term expires must sit out for at least a year before becoming eligible for reelection to the board. In order to bring new ideas into the deliberations of the old board, the 1971 agreement provided that one member would be replaced each year, beginning in 1972.

Partly as a result of Blanc Monroe's foresight and partly because young rebels have been heard, the Ochsner organization is flexible, a highly desirable quality in an age when the practice of medicine is changing. The founders were conservatives in matters of medical economics. Hines and his contemporaries had to swallow hard and adjust to government interference that was burdensome. New circumstances may force Porter and Riddick to take the institution into financial arrangements that Caldwell, Burns, *et al.*, would have found flabbergasting. Out of all the developments since 1955 one overriding fact has emerged: The Ochsner Institutions have been, are, and will be run by doctors.

CHAPTER EIGHT

Administrators: Surgeons and Laymen

In its first forty years the Ochsner Clinic has had five medical directors. The first doctor to have the title was Julius Lane Wilson. A highly regarded chest specialist, he joined the staff as a consultant in 1942, and became a full-time internist on May 1, 1946. Appointed director on April 14, 1950, Wilson had no illusions about "running the whole show." Instead, he recalled, "I considered myself a go-between, joining the partners and the staff." He never did penetrate the iron curtain, but his suggestion for creating the staff administrative advisory committee resulted in the first movement toward bringing employee-doctors into management.

When well into his eighties, Wilson still remembered an incident from his term as director when he had to answer the complaint of an irate patient who found on his bill an item for treatment by Thomas Findley, the chief internist. "I never saw any Dr. Findley," the man stormed. From the records Wilson learned that the patient had had a respiratory crisis after an operation, and Findley had resuscitated him while he was unconscious but had not gone to visit the man afterward. "He saved your life," Wilson explained.

Wilson yielded the directorship to Hiram W. Kostmayer on September 1, 1950, but remained in the internal medicine department until April 25, 1952, when he resigned to become a professor of medicine at the University of Pennsylvania. "It was a job that I wanted," he recalled many years later, but he conceded that his departure was partly prompted by the discord at Ochsner and the cloudy future.

Hiram W. Kostmayer's term as medical director was brief, but he put his stamp upon the office nonetheless. Kostmayer was a native New Orleanian, born on September 25, 1883. He received his bachelor of arts degree in 1904 and his doctor of medicine degree in 1909, both from Tulane University. He was the director of the Tulane graduate medical school and, in addition, served as acting dean of the medical school in 1932 and 1933 and again during the war years, 1942–1945.

Kostmayer was no yes-man, and he soon let the partners know it. One of the problems that arose during his tenure involved the anesthesiologists. Although they were on the clinic payroll, they did their work in the Foundation Hospital, and the hospital was sending out the bills for their services. This arrangement was contrary to the policy of the American Society of Anesthesiologists, and Guy Caldwell took it upon himself to remedy the situation. After conferring with George Bass Grant, head of the anesthesiology department, he worked out a solution with Blanc Monroe and reported it to Kostmayer.

The medical director was incensed. Directing copies to the other partners and Grant, he replied to Caldwell's memorandum with one of his own. "It seems to me," he wrote, "that the sending of this statement to me by you constitutes a very serious situation." It implied that Kostmayer had "been negligent in handling this matter and that it had to be pressed by you." Moreover, Caldwell had overstepped his authority in handling the matter as "between yourself and Dr. Grant on the one hand and Mr. Monroe on the other." Kostmayer reported that he had been discussing the problem and had hoped to arrive at an answer "which would not be obviously a subterfuge. . . . Under the circumstances," he concluded, "I wish to advise that I am filing the memorandum which you sent me and that I will take it up again for consideration only when and if it is presented to me through proper channels." Not many Ochsner doctors ever spoke so bluntly to one of the founders. Kostmayer had set a precedent for forthrightness that other medical directors would follow.

Kostmayer's term was abbreviated by his own choice. On May 15, 1951, in the midst of the staff turmoil, he notified the partners that he and his wife intended to move back to their home in Waveland, Mississippi, some time after August 1. He apologized for adding another problem in a troubled time and offered to commute by train. However, train schedules would not permit him to reach the clinic before 9:10 or

9:15 A.M., and he would have to leave by 2:40 or 2:45 P.M. "If you so desire," he said, "I will be very glad to do this either indefinitely if you believe that it will be satisfactory, or until you have found somebody to replace me as Director of the Clinic." Guy Caldwell took over the job first as acting medical director and then as director. Kostmayer lived for another thirty years, dying on December 3, 1981, at the age of ninety-eight.

The war was still being fought in both Europe and the Pacific in the summer of 1944 when a tall, emaciated (six-foot, one-inch, barely 120-pound) man wearing an army uniform with the insignia of a captain visited Alton Ochsner in the clinic building across the street from Touro Infirmary. Merrill Odom Hines was being discharged from the service because he was no longer physically able to attend to wounded men in the battle lines after he himself was felled by amebiasis in Italy. Now he wanted an opportunity to brush up on his surgery in preparation for entering private practice in Chattanooga. His meeting with Ochsner was a reunion. The surgeon had helped him get a Commonwealth Fund scholarship at the Tulane medical school and had taught him before he was graduated in 1936 as president of the senior class. Hines came onto the clinic staff a lamb; he turned into a lion.

Ochsner took him on as his assistant in general surgery, a prize apprenticeship, but it almost did Hines in. A prodigious worker himself, Ochsner took it for granted that his residents would check on patients before sunrise, then plunge into a round of activity that might last until midnight. He did not notice that after a few months Hines was showing distress. In attempting to treat his amebiasis in Italy, he had taken emetine, which damaged his heart. His ambition drove him on, but his weakened body rebelled. Finally, Thomas Findley noticed his plight. "What are you doing, trying to kill Hines?" the internist asked Ochsner. The contrite Ochsner reassigned Hines to less strenuous duties under another surgeon, Rawley M. Penick. It took several years, but eventually Hines's heart responded to the treatment of George E. Burch, Tulane cardiologist who served as a consultant on the clinic staff.

In fulfilling his obligation to the Commonwealth Fund for his scholarship, Hines had spent three years in Tylertown, Mississippi, where

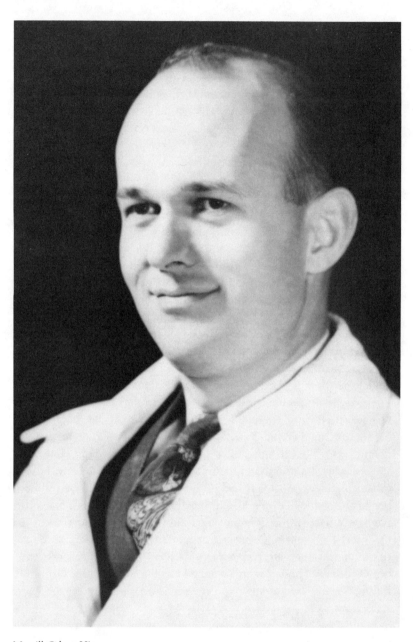

Merrill Odom Hines

he had to be a country doctor as well as a surgeon. He knew what it was to bring off a difficult delivery by lamplight in a sharecropper's cabin in a cotton field, with only a basin of hot water and the instruments in his doctor's bag to help him. It was a long jump from there to a gleaming operating room in a New Orleans hospital, with trays of scalpels and scissors at hand and a skilled team of doctors, nurses, and technicians in support. In Tylertown, one on one with every patient who sought his ministrations, Hines learned the compassion that guided him throughout his subsequent career. There was more to medicine than money and fame.

At the clinic he found what he was looking for and abandoned his plan for practicing in Chattanooga. "Something tremendous is happening here, and I want to be a part of it," he told Alton Ochsner. Hines suggested that he develop a colon and rectal surgery department. In August, 1945, he went to the Mayo Clinic to spend three months studying under the surgeons who had pioneered in the methods by which general surgeons performed colon and rectal procedures. Upon his return he took over the work that fell within the area of his expertise, and Ochsner was in business as the second clinic with such a department. The Cleveland Clinic was third.

Later Hines, as a part-time teacher at Tulane, persuaded Robert Bernhard, the Charity Hospital director, to supply a big basement room at Charity for a proctology department. Hines and Patrick Hanley, who had joined the Ochsner staff, hung up curtains to divide the room into four areas so both could make proctoscopic examinations simultaneously. They had to make do with whatever furniture they could scrounge. Once, in the middle of an examination a makeshift table overturned, dumping the patient onto the floor and breaking a nurse's foot. The persuasive Hines talked the patient into getting back onto the table.

Proctology and colon surgery became an independent specialty in 1949. As a leader in the field, Hines was elected president of the American Proctologic Society, now the American Society of Colon and Rectal Surgeons, and also served as president of the American Board of Colon and Rectal Surgery.

Hines was only beginning to emerge as an influential member of the staff in the early 1950s, the uneasy period of conflict between the founders and the hired professional staff. He had not yet attained professonal stature to equal that of Dean Echols, Rawley Penick, or William R. Arrowsmith, for instance. But having tied his career to the fortunes of the clinic, he was determined that the organization would not break up in discord. As president of the foundation hospital staff, he told the partners that the iron curtain behind which they operated was one of the reasons for the strain and counseled better communications. His was a voice of moderation, in contrast to the shrillness that marked the complaints of some dissident staff members.

Hines became involved in the management of the clinic in 1954 with his appointment as assistant medical director to work under Guy Caldwell's supervision. In 1960, as Caldwell approached retirement age, Hines succeeded him as medical director. It was Hines's lot to preside during the transition period when one founder after another reached the seventieth-birthday milestone that ended active participation in clinic and foundation affairs. Control was being passed along to the heirs. The second generation had to prove its worth, and Hines, as titular leader of the clinic and president, later chairman, of the foundation trustees was thrust into the job with the most responsibility.

His fifteen years as medical director and ten years as president or chairman proved to be a prosperous and productive era for clinic and foundation. Patients came in increasing numbers for diagnosis and treatment by a medical staff that was multiplying in size. The challenge to Hines, backed up by the old-timers who controlled the board of management, was to inspire the newcomers to practice with the zeal and skill that the founders had demanded. Highly qualified department and section chiefs were essential, and Hines willingly saw to it that some men were attracted by incomes that exceeded his own salary.

On the foundation side, the Jefferson Highway plant was brought up to its present capacity. Death had removed J. Blanc Monroe and Theodore Brent from the board of trustees. But Richard W. Freeman stepped into the breach, taking an active hand in foundation affairs. He and Hines made an effective management team. Associates called them "Mr. Outside" and "Mr. Inside."

It was during Hines's administration that the founders and some of the older staff doctors finally abandoned their hopes for a merger of the Ochsner Medical Institutions and Tulane University. When final negotiations bogged down, the Tulane medical faculty moved ahead with plans for a group practice of its own, and the school built its own teaching hospital. Informal talk about starting an Ochsner medical school never reached a serious stage.

Oddly, it was the old-timers, the ones who had tried unsuccessfully to work out an accommodation with Tulane, who were the most enthusiastic when the subject of an affiliation came up again in 1965. They could envision benefits to Ochsner's fellowship training program resulting from a merger. More important, they had seen federal government appropriations for medical research increase in twenty years from $32 million to $500 million. But the signals from Washington seemed to say that almost all of the money would be channeled through university medical schools. Tulane, too, would benefit from a merger, gaining a ready-made teaching hospital, financial support provided by a share of the receipts from the clinic, and dozens of part-time instructors and researchers from the Ochsner staff.

Discussions grew out of chats between Charles C. Sprague, dean of the Tulane medical school, and Hines, a Tulane alumnus. The first formal meeting was held at Tulane on February 1, 1965. Participating doctors on the medical school side were Sprague, George E. Burch, Oscar Creech, and Robert G. Heath, all department heads. Guy Caldwell accompanied Hines to the session.

Before long the foundation trustees, the clinic board of management, the Tulane board of administrators, and the executive faculty of the medical school all were drawn into the negotiations. Tulane obtained a $250,000 grant from the Commonwealth Fund to finance a study of the proposal. Although no plan ever won the approval of all participants, a preliminary arrangement was drawn up. Under its provisions, the Ochsner Clinic partnership would have been dissolved and reorganized as the Ochsner Clinic Association. Tulane faculty members would have had the privilege of buying membership in the association and practicing in the group. The Ochsner Foundation would have deeded the hospital and its other properties to Tulane. The Clinic Association would then have leased its facilities from Tulane, paying a proportion of its revenue. Association doctors who volunteered would have been paid by Tulane for part-time teaching or research activities.

The clinic partnership debated the advantages and disadvantages over a period of months, and founders and senior staff members were outspoken advocates. Among those who raised questions was Walter S. Culpepper, who warned that Tulane would gain much from a wedding, whereas the dowry that the clinic would have to pay was "quite handsome, with few advantages in exchange." He said members of the Ochsner staff had worked hard to build up a "tremendous medical group with a high reputation," but the merger would mean "inviting a like number of comparative outsiders to partake of the fruits of their hard labor." A vital issue, never resolved to the satisfaction of the Ochsner staff, was the question of whether the clinic departments would be headed by Ochsner doctors or Tulane faculty. Hines said the Tulane negotiators first assigned the posts to Ochsner clinicians but later backed off. As talks continued, increasing opposition developed in the Tulane faculty.

While the matter simmered, late in 1966, Hines and Edgar J. Saux went to Washington and discovered a drastic change in the government's policy concerning federal aid for medicine. The thinking now was that university-affiliated medical centers treated less than 1 percent of the nation's population, and the government intended to direct its support to facilities where most patients received care. It was on this point that the merger lost most of its attractiveness to the Ochsner partnership. Representatives of both sides agreed at a meeting on December 19, 1966, that the project was not financially feasible. Without the affiliation, Ochsner continued to build up its facilities and enlarge its activities. Tulane also was able to finance a medical center and embark on a faculty group practice. Would the institutions have prospered even more had they wed? Perhaps yes, perhaps no. But there was a basic incompatibility they would have had to overcome. Ochsner's primary reason for being is to provide clinical care; Tulane's is teaching.

The debate had just begun when, on February 11, 1965, Merrill Hines secured board of management approval of a $100,000 donation of clinic funds to Tulane's Forward Drive. Some partners, particularly those who had graduated from other schools, opposed the gift, and when a new partnership agreement was adopted in 1971, it forbade donations by the board of more than $2,500 to any organization other than the Alton Ochsner Medical Foundation. Larger gifts to others now require a vote of the entire partnership.

It was under Hines and later Frank Riddick that the medical directorship became the powerful position it is today. These two consolidated the influence Guy Caldwell, as a founder, had brought to the post. Merrill Hines's instincts told him to meet every problem head-on, and the record shows few, if any, times when he ducked a confrontation. He spoke his mind, frequently bruising egos, but most of the staff physicians and lay employees recognized that he was a disciplinarian because he was dedicated to the best interests of the institutions. Even so, he brought on much grumbling by advocating generous contributions by the clinic to the foundation.

Always respectful, even diffident, when he was dealing with one of the founding partners, especially Ochsner, Hines discovered himself in a dilemma as May 1, 1967, approached. By clinic rules, Ochsner on that day would become ineligible to perform surgery. He had turned seventy on May 4, 1966. The rules provide that a surgeon can operate until the last day of the fiscal year in which his seventieth birthday falls. For Ochsner this meant he could keep going until four days before his seventy-first birthday. The vigorous surgeon, for whose services patient demand continued as brisk as ever, was not ready to retire. Hines went to see him and reminded him that the day was approaching. "I won't quit," Ochsner responded. Hines waited a few days to see whether the surgeon would relent. When Ochsner showed no signs of doing so, Hines paid him another visit on a Sunday morning. He acknowledged Ochsner's leadership in surgery, but he said, Ochsner had concurred when the retirement rule was adopted years earlier. "If you don't retire, we'll tear up the agreement," Hines said, "but I want you to know that if that happens, I have no alternative but to resign myself."

"God damn it," Ochsner blurted, "you get out of here. I'll quit."

Specific terms for Ochsner's retirement were worked out at a series of Sunday morning meetings of the founders. Ochsner could continue to occupy his office in the clinic. He could treat but not operate on patients who asked to see him, and he could keep 95 percent of the fees collected. He also would receive a pension of $18,000 a year, the retirement income for all of the founders under a formula in the clinic pension plan. On his final day in an operating room, on April 30, 1967, Ochsner put on a show to end all doubts about whether he could have continued. He performed thirteen surgical procedures.

A surgeon is figuratively naked when he approaches a patient on an operating table in a big metropolitan hospital. He has no way of concealing professional shortcomings from the knowledgeable doctors and nurses who make up an operative team. Reputation, personal connections, bluster—nothing can cover up a lack of judgment and skill that becomes glaringly obvious to the initiated. Inevitably, there are whispers and remarks in surgeons' lounges and nursing stations. The word spreads throughout the hospital.

A situation such as this confronted Hines not long after he became medical director. A surgeon who had been trained in prestigious institutions and who appeared to be highly qualified joined the staff. He had known many of the partners for years and was personally popular. In a short while he became influential in clinic affairs. But at the same time his performance in the operating room failed to meet the institutions' standards. After a while, internists were referring patients to outsiders in order to avoid sending them to him for surgery. Some operating room nurses were reluctant to work with him. On the Ochsner campus the turn of events was far from secret.

"Somebody had to act, and I knew it was I," Hines related afterward. The medical director suggested the man take on a nonsurgical assignment, such as head of research and education, but the latter balked. The professional personnel committee investigated and found deficiencies in the surgeon's performance. He threatened to sue for libel.

Finally Hines forced a showdown. He obtained signatures from an overwhelming number of the clinic's doctors, who said they would vote to oust the surgeon from the partnership under a bylaw that provides for expulsion by three-fourths' majority. The man resigned.

"It was the most difficult decision I ever had to make, and at the same time was the most important one," Hines said. "I didn't see how we could continue in business if we allowed an unqualified surgeon to operate, no matter who he was. When we admit a patient to our Clinic or Hospital, we must guarantee that he will be in competent hands."

It was part of the medical director's job to see to it that those who could not meet the standards did not stay on. Hines arranged for more than one doctor to be discharged. There was an internist, for example, who failed to keep patient records up to date and who would not write the obligatory follow-up letters to doctors who had referred patients. Once, while this doctor was on vacation, Hines found a stack of unopened mail in his office. In another instance, a highly recommended surgeon was discharged because he could not be located at times when he was scheduled to be on call.

Hines and the FBI-agent-turned-administrator, Edgar J. Saux, proved adept at detective work when it was required to solve clinic problems. They scored their most spectacular triumph in a mystery involving one of the surgery subspecialties. Upon entering his office a staff doctor used to flip a switch that turned on a light at the reception desk in the waiting room and notified the receptionists that he was on duty. Hines began to receive complaints that the light of one of the surgeons was frequently off when he was due to be at work. When the medical director confronted the man about what appeared to be unauthorized absences, the latter insisted he had been in his office. Hines and Saux set to work. Saux rigged up a photographic device in the office and waited. Before long he and Hines had the answer—clear pictures of another surgeon in the department bending down behind a desk to reach the switch and turn off his colleague's light on the receptionist's panel. His motive apparently was to have patients referred to him in the presumed absence of the other man. His denials sputtered out when Hines showed him the photographs.

No one, not even any of the founders, was as fiercely devoted to the Ochsner Institutions as Merrill Hines became. For years, he worked a fourteen-hour day, seven days a week. In 1980, as the day approached when he would have to retire because of age, he was miserable at the prospect of an existence away from Ochsner. The trustees of the foundation made an exception for him. They created the unique position of honorary chairman of the board, allowing him to continue fund raising and planning. No one else, not even Alton Ochsner, was given such a concession.

But the climax of Hines's career came in 1983 with his selection as the forty-sixth recipient of the Distinguished Service Award of the

American Medical Association. The award, created in 1938, is the most coveted honor given in the Western Hemisphere to a practitioner of the healing arts. Annually, the AMA recognizes only one doctor for exceptional contributions to medicine, either in scientific achievement or in furthering the delivery of health care or both. Hines was a worthy recipient. Not only did he pioneer in the emergence of colon and rectal surgery as a specialty, but he played a prominent part in the development of the Ochsner Medical Institutions and he was an influence in AMA councils for many years. The award represented a triumph for Ochsner as well as for Hines, for he was the fourth surgeon with ties to the clinic to earn this distinction. Only the Mayo Clinic can claim an equal number of former or present associates who have won the AMA's premier prize. The first man ever to receive the prize was Rudolph Matas. Michael DeBakey, who joined the clinic at the outset, was chosen in 1959 after he had moved to Houston. Alton Ochsner received the prize in 1967 and regarded it as one of the highlights of his extraordinary career.

The Ochsner Institutions are staffed with excellent doctors, it is true, but many lay people have also devoted themselves to its success. One particularly devoted layman, the only one ever proposed for partnership in the Ochsner Clinic, was Edgar J. Saux, who succeeded Junius Underwood as business manager on September 14, 1951. By 1957, when the partnership was enlarged, Saux had won the approbation of Guy Caldwell and the other founders. Caldwell put Saux's name on the list of men selected to join in the proprietorship. J. Blanc Monroe scratched it off, on the grounds that the partnership should be confined to physicians and surgeons. With the backing of others, Caldwell tried again, but Monroe was adamant. Finally, rather than become a source of contention, Saux asked Caldwell to yield. Over the years until his retirement in 1980, Saux sat in on the highest councils of clinic and foundation. His title was changed to administrator and then to administrative director.

The former special agent of the Federal Bureau of Investigation was office manager of the New Orleans *Item* when Caldwell interviewed him. "I didn't know a thing about medicine," he recalls. "Dr. LeJeune told me he was an otolaryngologist, and I said, 'Hell, I can't even pronounce the word.' Medical terms floored me, but I had four children

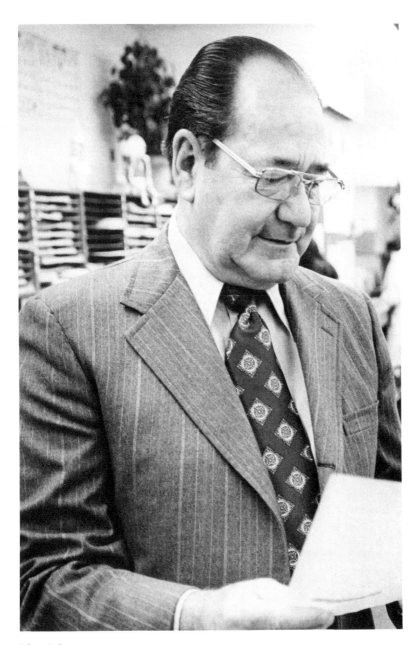

Edgar J. Saux

and I knew what a B.M. was." Caldwell explained that the big problem was employee relations, damaged during Underwood's regime. Saux was well suited to improving that situation. Slow to scold but quick of wit, he soon lifted clinic morale.

His biggest challenge was orchestrating the move in 1963 from the original clinic building at Prytania and Aline to the new building on the Jefferson Highway campus. It was reported at the time to be the biggest moving operation yet carried out in New Orleans. The old clinic was closed after the last patient left on a Thursday afternoon. An endless line of trucks began hauling furniture, equipment, and thousands of envelopes of patient records that had to be put at the fingertips of library personnel so that any one of them could be located immediately at the request of a physician. There were only two entrances, the front and back doors. If a truck got out of line, there was no place for it to unload. Nurses and receptionists put on jeans or old clothes and worked around the clock.

After visiting other clinics around the country, Saux decided to change the unit control system for receiving patients to a plan in which a nursing station on each floor directed the flow. He compiled a book with detailed instructions.

At eight o'clock on Monday morning the doors were opened. Confusion ensued. "Nothing was working but the clock, and it was thirty minutes late." Records became jammed in the serpentine six-story chute. An elevator got stuck between the fourth and fifth floors and trapped ten women, most of them employees. Saux directed another elevator alongside. He climbed over the top, lowered a chair through a trapdoor for the women to stand on, and lifted them one after another to the top, where they could step over to the other car.

Old nurses were in tears from frustration while Saux kept insisting order would be restored. "I was scared silly, and kept praying, 'Lord, make it work.'" Edgar Burns went to Saux's office. "Ed, it's impossible," he groaned. "Just wait, it'll be all right," the business manager replied. And finally, everything fell into place.

Gifts from patients had provided Alton Ochsner with the trappings for a handsome office during the time the clinic had operated the general surgery department in Brent House. He transferred the furniture to his new office and started with an impressive layout. Meanwhile, the board of management had decided that the other partners would have to make do with their furniture from the old clinic. The offices of the others therefore looked shabby in comparison with Ochsner's. Some of LeJeune's friends and patients twitted him, "I thought you said there were five equal partners." Mrs. LeJeune informed Saux that her husband was "hurt and embarrassed." She set about arranging a "little gem" for LeJeune, and the board voted to allow each founder any kind of office he wanted. Burns had a window cut in the wall in order to see the river. Tyrone told Saux he wanted nothing special and would keep his office as it was "to show how badly I am treated around here."

When Saux retired, on April 30, 1980, Francis F. (Mel) Manning assumed the title administrative director. Manning had joined the administrative staff in 1964 as associate administrator and moved up to administrator when Saux was appointed administrative director in 1972. He is the author of *Group Practice Management.*

PART II

Ochsner's Expands

CHAPTER NINE

The Patients

The patients who flocked to Ochsner after the lull of 1950–1951 looked for and received the expert care they had come to expect. The thirty years since the mid-fifties have seen more advances in medical treatment than ever before. Ochsner has remained in the vanguard and its patients—black and white, rich and poor—have benefitted.

Clint W. Murchison avoided doctors, and if he had not been affected with the miseries in February, 1956, he would never have consented to stop off at the Ochsner Foundation Hospital while he was enroute from his island in the Bahamas to his ranch in Texas. Alton Ochsner, who arranged the admission, knew instinctively that A. Seldon "Sam" Mann was just the internist to assign to the case. Thus began a fortuitous chapter in the annals of the Ochsner Institutions.

In the years before his retirement, Sam Mann was one of the busiest staff members the clinic ever had. A husky, low-key North Carolinian, he knew how to get the most out of the art of medicine. "Listen to your patients," he replied to a trainee who asked his advice. Mann took time to listen. He was sympathetic, forgave occasional lapses from the regimens he prescribed, and was candid and forthcoming in his discussions with patients. He won Murchison's confidence from the first day.

After undergoing tests at the hospital, the Texan went to the old clinic building to hear the results. He found himself seated in Mann's cubbyhole office, which had barely enough room to accommodate himself, Mann, and Ochsner, who sat in on the conference. "It's a damn shame you have to work in a place like this," Murchison commented. "You need a new building." His interest and generosity eventually were major factors in the construction of the clinic building which now abuts the hospital on the Ochsner campus.

Mann became the Texas tycoon's principal health consultant. Sometimes Murchison would come to New Orleans for tests. He looked into the possibilities of acquiring a private suite in the hospital, and when that plan proved unworkable, he considered building a penthouse atop Brent House where he and his relatives and business associates could stay in seclusion—and enjoy a magnificent view of the Mississippi River—while they were receiving medical attention. Construction problems finally ruled out the penthouse, however, and Murchison and members of his circle ended up using the regular facilities.

Often over a thirteen-year period Murchison sent his luxuriously appointed airplane, a converted DC3 christened the *Flying Ginnie* in honor of his wife, Virginia, to New Orleans to pick up Mann, and sometimes other Ochsner doctors. Murchison's personal crew would fly Mann and whoever was with him to the Texan's ranch at Athens, Texas, to his secluded ranch in the mountains of Mexico, or to his island in the Gulf of Mexico near Tampico. "Bring your little black bag," Murchison would instruct, and Mann would examine his patient and prescribe for him before going hunting or fishing.

One visit to the Mexican ranch resulted in a medical first. Ochsner had obtained newly developed equipment that allowed the signals of electrocardiography to be transmitted through a regular telephone connection to be recorded and interpreted at a hospital or clinic. Mann in Mexico collaborated with Charles B. Moore in New Orleans in checking Murchison's heartbeat. It was the first time the procedure had been used as an international transmission. Late in the process, the telephone operator broke the connection. "She must have thought we were spies," Mann comments. Three weeks later the procedure was used by others in a trans-Atlantic reading involving the motion picture actor Edward G. Robinson in London.

Murchison habitually arose early and began making telephone calls to the managers of the enterprises in his business empire. Once, in Athens, Texas, when Mann was a houseguest, he wandered into the room where his host was talking. Murchison looked up. "I think I am going to buy a football team," he told the doctor. And he did—the Dallas Cowboys of the National Football League.

On another occasion at the Athens ranch, a fellow guest, Perry R. Bass, asked Mann, "Will you go to Fort Worth with me and help me get Uncle Sid to a hospital? He is sick and he won't do anything about it." Uncle Sid was Sid W. Richardson, an oil and gas developer whose wealth rivaled that of his close friend Murchison. Mann, who had met Richardson socially but never treated him, flew with Bass to Fort Worth and examined Richardson. "You need to be in a hospital," Mann told him. "Nobody can help you unless you are. Come on down to the Ochsner hospital now. I'm ready to go with you." They made the flight at once, and Richardson became Mann's patient for the rest of his life. He too would send his personal plane to pick up Mann, sometimes meeting him at his hideaway, St. Joseph Island, off the Texas coast. Mann recalls visiting Richardson once as the latter was completing a session with his auditors. "All I owe now is $50 million," he told the physician.

Like Murchison, Richardson was fond of Alton Ochsner, and sometimes invited him to come with Mann on flights to Texas. St. Joseph Island, a low-lying range dotted by clumps of bushes, is a nesting place for quail. Richardson had a jeep built with special seats on each side of the radiator. His technique was to assign a hunter to each seat. A driver, sometimes his airplane pilot, Don Beeler, would drive the jeep up to a clump of bushes and race the engine. Out would fly birds at point-blank range for the occupants of the special seats. Richardson did not like to see birds wounded. He wanted them dispatched on the first shot. One day Ochsner, riding in a hunter's seat, soon proved he was no marksman. "Doctor," Richardson asked, "what is the first thing you do when you are about to begin a surgical operation?" "Why, I scrub and put on surgical gloves," Ochsner replied. Richardson interrupted and turned to Beeler, who was driving the jeep. "Look around and see if you've got any surgical gloves with you," he directed.

The Texas millionaires Mann treated were well able to pay the fees and to give lavish gifts as well. Mann sometimes received boxes of grapefruit, boots, and even an automobile was once delivered to his home. But Ochsner was not founded to take care of only wealthy people. In the nine fiscal years beginning in 1974 the Ochsner Foundation Hospital provided free services with a total value of $4,208,586 to patients who could not pay and were not covered by government or private insurance. The charity work far exceeded Ochsner's commitment to serve indigent patients in return for the funds it has received for building facilities under terms of the Hill-Burton Act. It carried out provisions of the foundation charter, which was drawn up before Medicare and Medicaid removed thousands of persons from dependence on free care.

In 1971 a group of area residents filed suit against a number of New Orleans hospitals, including Ochsner, contending that the institutions had not fulfilled Hill-Burton requirements to provide substantial charity care for the indigent. Federal judges ruled that each of the defendant hospitals would have to make available every year for ten years free services equal to 10 percent of the total amount of Hill-Burton funds it had received. Ochsner's obligation on this basis was $223,000 a year. Although by far most of the persons who seek medical services at Ochsner have funds to pay their way or are covered by insurance, nobody is turned away from the emergency room because of a lack of money. Patients are given immediate treatment. Some are later transferred to Charity Hospital, which is operated by the state of Louisiana to take care of the uninsured indigent.

Similarly, blacks have never been denied treatment at clinic or hospital. Four of the five founders were southerners, but whatever prejudices they may have had did not prevent the clinic from accepting black patients from the beginning, and the same policy applied to Splinter Village and later to the Ochsner Foundation Hospital. In the custom of most of the New Orleans medical community, the institutions did not actively seek black patients, but neither did the staff turn them away when they sought appointments.

Before Congress passed civil rights legislation in 1963, however, few blacks came to Ochsner. Records show that from 1956 until 1961 the numbers of black patients treated in the hospital each year were only 38, 75, 75, 59, 50, and 79. In 1962 the board encouraged the staff to send patients who required hospitalization to the Flint Goodridge Hospital, a black institution, and to the Sara Mayo Hospital, which sought black patronage. During one period, blacks were designated as "special patients," and during another, "A patients." Efforts were made to make them inconspicuous. When the new clinic building opened in 1963, the waiting rooms were divided by lines of potted plants, and the board of management directed that some restrooms be labeled "colored."

But when civil rights legislation was passed, Merrill Hines told the board of management and the trustees that Ochsner would comply. In 1964 he and Edgar Saux made the rounds of the clinic waiting rooms and took down the "colored" signs from the restrooms. The Brent House hotel and restaurants were formally integrated as well. In 1964 the trustees certified that the hospital was in conformity with requirements of the Hill-Burton Act that black patients not be discriminated against. Not until 1978 was the first black staff doctor, radiologist Joseph B. Prejean, hired, however. Cherryll L. Blythe, assigned to the emergency room in 1981, was the second.

As the United States moved ahead toward a more just society, Ochsner doctors advanced the practice of medicine. The 1970s might be called the decade of cardiology, for during those years, knowledge of how to repair the human heart burgeoned. But it was in 1967 that Christiaan Barnard of South Africa performed the operation that awed and alarmed the lay public: He transplanted a human heart.

The wave of heart transplants reported in headlines around the world made it evident that sooner or later Ochsner surgeons would be faced with a situation in which the new procedure might save a life. Alton Ochsner's son John assembled a team, and each member learned his or her role in a series of practices with animals. Once Ochsner was satisfied that his team was ready, the waiting began. The difficulty of obtaining suitable hearts is a barrier that will always limit the number of human transplants. An organ must be taken from the donor's body immediately upon death, before it deteriorates. Pure chance governs the availability of a heart, and there is no recourse save to keep a patient alive until a donor, usually one who has been injured in an accident, dies.

On Christmas Day, 1969, the curtain rose on the first scene. William I. Taylor of Metairie was admitted to the Ochsner Foundation Hospital for treatment of congestive heart failure, the result of arteriosclerotic coronary artery disease. Tests showed his heart to be too ravaged to respond to bypass surgery or to be kept pumping for very long with drugs. Surgeons and cardiologists explained to Taylor and his wife the alternative of a transplant, making clear that it was an untried operation in Louisiana and outlining the risks. Although the mechanics of changing hearts had been mastered and operating room mortality was low, the number of long-term survivals was small because the human body tends to reject the intrusion of foreign tissue. The rejection process can be controlled with drugs, but these lower resistance to disease, making a patient vulnerable to fatal infections. Taylor and his wife elected to take the gamble.

Early on Thursday morning, January 8, 1970, John L. Ochsner was awakened at his home. A suitable donor was dying. Ochsner gave instructions for the transplant team to be assembled, and headed for the hospital. At her home in uptown New Orleans, Pamela Weiss, a suture nurse, had a telephone call. "Hurry on out; we have a donor. Don't say anything to anybody," she was told.

A thirty-six-year-old woman was wheeled into Room No. 7 of the surgical suite. Immediately after she died, Robert D. Bloodwell removed her heart. Next door, in Room No. 8, Ochsner had attached Taylor to the heart-lung apparatus and opened his chest. Then he sent Pamela Weiss to bring the donor heart. Bloodwell handed her a basin in which it lay, still throbbing.

"Come on, give it to me," Ochsner ordered, and Weiss lifted the organ out of the basin. The surgeon, who by now had excised Taylor's heart, inserted the substitute heart into the chest and connected the arteries and veins. An electric shock set the new heart to beating regularly. Ochsner disconnected the heart-lung machine and closed the chest. The suspense seemed to be over.

Then developed a problem without reported precedent in the scores of other heart transplants done in the United States and abroad. The new heart faltered in its functioning. Ochsner realized that Taylor had a complete tricuspid insufficiency. A heart that had given the donor no trouble was now malfunctioning.

What should have been the denouement of the drama became the climax instead. Ochsner moved swiftly. He put Taylor back onto heart-lung machine circulation, reopened the chest through the incision he had made for the transplant, and repaired the faulty tricuspid valve with valvuloplasty. In a period of less than two hours Ochsner had performed on the same patient not only a heart transplant but also open-heart surgery, an unheard-of combination. The repaired heart worked well, and after installing a pacemaker Ochsner sent Taylor to the recovery room.

As she completed her follow-up duties and started home, Pamela Weiss was surprised to hear a radio station broadcast a news report of the transplant.

Taylor was walking by the time he left the hospital, but the immunosuppressive drugs given to prevent rejection of the heart left him without adequate defense against pneumonia. He died on May 4, 1970. The heart was found at autopsy to be in good shape, and there was no indication that the rejection phenomenon had begun.

Subsequent patients who have inquired about transplants have been referred to Stanford University, where most of the procedures now take place and where surgeons have perfected a sensitive biopsy test for signs of rejection and thus are enabled to prescribe the immunosuppressive drugs sparingly.

In a letter to Cardiologist Philip Bowers, Mrs. Taylor expressed no regrets over the decision for a transplant. "The doctors and nurses were wonderful to my husband, my children and myself during our trying times. They were both patient and helpful. You gave my husband a few more months of life. I know we were all hoping he would have a prolonged and useful life but we all knew it was experimental and I feel in my heart you all tried with untiring energy. I know Ochsner Hospital some day will find the secret to a prolonged heart transplant."

Not all heart surgery is as risky as the transplant. Over a twenty-month period in the middle 1970s, Ochsner heart surgeons John Ochsner and Noel L. Mills performed 322 consecutive arterial bypass procedures without a single operative death. Their record was a milestone in the development of the bypass as an acceptable method of relieving angina pectoris and improving the quality of life for patients whose clogged arteries cut off the flow of blood to the heart. For nearly two decades some cardiologists opposed the open-heart operation as a risky procedure that provided results no better than they could obtain with drugs and bed rest.

The surgical objective is to restore the supply of blood reaching heart muscles by providing detours around the coronary arteries that have become blocked by the disease process known as atherosclerosis. Substitute blood vessels are grafted into the circulatory system, bypassing from one to as many as six arteries, while a patient is maintained on the heart-lung apparatus.

Ochsner and Mills used meticulous techniques to achieve their results. They took advantage of magnification for precise surgery, closely monitored patients' vital signs, worked swiftly in order to depend upon the heart-lung apparatus as briefly as possible. When feasible they used a patient's own internal mammary arteries for grafts. When they substituted a saphenous vein from the patient's leg, they handled it gently to avoid clot-forming injury to the tissue. They demanded that patients who smoked give up cigarettes and refused to operate on any who balked.

By the early 1980s opposition to bypass was crumbling. By this time the operative mortality at Ochsner was less than 1 percent and approaching .5 percent. Paradoxically, the operation was so successful that some patients had to have it repeated. After five to eight years, the grafts installed during the original surgery themselves became atherosclerotic and needed replacing. The patients would not have been alive long enough for this to happen, of course, had the first bypass not been successful.

Still, the cardiologists at Ochsner sought ways to deal with blocked arteries that would avoid the harmful effects of the heart-lung machine and the other disadvantages of open-heart surgery. In October, 1980, Gerald Piltz, a certified public accountant from Biloxi, Mississippi, entered the Ochsner Foundation Hospital in the expectation of undergoing heart bypass surgery to relieve the pain of angina. His wife, Flo, had benefitted from the same operation two years earlier and he was hopeful of good results, although he did not look forward to an open-heart operation.

After angiography confirmed the blockage of one of Piltz's coronary arteries, Charles Lynn Skelton, cardiologist, went to see him. "Maybe you are lucky," Skelton told him. "If you want to be a guinea pig, we may be able to solve your problem without surgery." And he explained that the angiogram indicated that Piltz was a good candidate for percutaneous transluminal angioplasty. What he proposed to do was to use a newly developed balloon catheter to open up the clogged section of a coronary artery and restore the flow of blood. Skelton warned that a risk was involved, and pointed out that the first attempt at Ochsner had been a failure. "I don't have anything to lose," responded Piltz. "Let's go."

Skelton made a tiny incision in an artery in Piltz's upper leg and inserted a sleeve catheter. With the aid of fluoroscopy, he threaded the catheter through the artery and into the heart to the exact location where the vessel was obstructed. Then through this outer catheter he introduced a smaller catheter which has a tiny ballon at the end. When the balloon emerged from the sleeve, Skelton pressed on the plunger of a small pump and forced air through the catheter to inflate it. This enlarged the artery, and when the balloon was deflated and the catheters withdrawn, blood coursed through to the heart.

Two months later, Piltz was back at the hospital. In his caution, Skelton had not inflated the balloon enough and the artery clogged up again. Surgeon John Ochsner watched as Skelton repeated the procedure. "Pop the hell out of it," Ochsner directed, and Skelton did. This time the obstruction was completely cleared. Nearly two years later the artery became occluded again, in a different section, and for the third time Skelton did his act. Since then, Piltz, who was fifty-five years old when the procedure first was used on him, has been without pain and without restriction on his activity. He found the angioplasty, performed with only a local anesthetic, to be virtually painless.

Skelton had become interested in angioplasty during the late 1970s. In January, 1980, he went to Zurich, Switzerland, to watch Professor Andreas Gruntzig demonstrate the procedure. On July 22, 1980, Skelton was ready for the first clinical trial at Ochsner. Ten minutes after he withdrew the catheter the patient, a Metairie resident, experienced severe chest pains. He was taken immediately to an operating room, where he underwent successful bypass surgery. Angioplasty is done at Ochsner only when a standby operating room is open and when heart surgeons are on hand to do a bypass if necessary. Of the first 280 cases at Ochsner, there were no deaths. Three-fourths of the procedures brought satisfactory results. Fewer than twenty patients required emergency operations. About forty others were not helped by angioplasty and later underwent elective surgery.

Skelton said the procedure has been proven a safe and effective way of postponing or even avoiding bypass. In late 1982 it still was used only when one of the three main coronary arteries was blocked, but

Skelton predicted that it would be successfully applied in the future when two or even three arteries are occluded.

For the Ochsner Institutions, angioplasty is good medicine but poor business. A patient need stay in the hospital only three days, and the fees and other charges are only one-third or less of the total cost of bypass surgery. But Ochsner physicians are looking for better ways to treat their patients. Sometimes surgery is the best or even the only available way to restore a patient to health; sometimes there is another way.

On April 8, 1975, a pioneering Ochsner team introduced a device with which a hole in the heart can be closed without surgery. The King-Mills cardiac umbrella won for its inventors, Terry D. King and Noel L. Mills, the Young Inventors Award of the American Pediatric Society. When King, a pediatric cardiologist, joined the Ochsner Clinic staff he discovered that he and Mills, a heart surgeon, had independently been toying with the idea of mending such natal anomalies as atrial and ventrical septal defects with the help of heart catheters. After working together for three years they demonstrated on animals a device that worked.

The doctors decided to make the first clinical trial of their invention on seventeen-year-old Suzette Marie Creppel of Metairie, who had been handicapped since birth by a secundum atrial septal defect, an opening in the wall that divides the chambers of the heart. The only repair previously available would have involved placing her on a heart-lung machine and opening the heart, a major surgical procedure.

Instead, with the assistance of Nurse Sandra L. Thompson, Mills and King first measured the hole in the heart wall by introducing a balloon catheter into a femoral vein in the patient's right leg and guiding it through the inferior vena cava into the heart. By deflating the balloon until the catheter passed through the defect, they could estimate the dimensions of the hole. A surgical team stood by until the measurement indicated that the defect was suitable for closure with the umbrella. Otherwise, the team would have performed the conventional open-heart operation.

Now came the first human test of the King-Mills umbrella. A capsule containing two tiny closed dacron umbrellas was attached to a catheter made up of outer and inner tubes, through one of which each of the umbrellas could be opened. Watching the progress through fluoroscopy, the doctors guided the catheter through the same veins. Manipulated through the catheter, one of the umbrellas was opened to its one-and-a-half-inch diameter on one side of the wall. The other was expanded on the other side, and the two locked together. The opening was sealed. The catheter was withdrawn, and ninety minutes after Suzette had entered the laboratory she was taken back to her hospital room. Seventy-two hours later her swollen heart had shrunk by a third. The disabling shunt was closed.

Suzette, at seventeen, was a young heart patient but not by any means the youngest. On July 27, 1974, John L. Ochsner implanted a heart pacemaker in the youngest patient ever. The nine-pound, two-ounce recipient was only eighteen hours old.

At birth in the station hospital at Keesler Air Force Base, Biloxi, Mississippi, Jason Haines showed distress. Major Luther Williams found that his heartbeat was only half the normal rate and diagnosed a complete congenital heart block. The air force doctor used an external pacemaker to keep the heart beating and accompanied the baby on a hundred-mile ambulance ride to the Ochsner center.

Terry D. King, pediatric cardiologist, prepared the child for surgery. Ochsner found that the temporary pacemaker was not working. He installed an infant-sized permanent pacemaker into the tiny body, and the heart responded immediately.

Two years later Ochsner implanted a replacement lithium pacemaker. Jason had developed into a healthy baby, with no problems other than the failure of the natural mechanism to maintain a normal heartbeat. An anomaly known as patent ductus arteriosus had corrected itself spontaneously.

Ochsner Foundation Hospital contains the best equipped neonatal intensive care unit in the Deep South. It serves Lousiana and all or part of seven other southern states. Every year, more than five hundred seriously ill babies, most of them born prematurely, are transported in airplane or surface ambulances to the special Ochsner unit, where they receive expert care.

Twins—Tram, four pounds, fourteen ounces, and Mollie, three pounds, fifteen ounces—were born to Bert Jones, quarterback of the Baltimore Colts professional football team, and his wife in Saint Francis Hospital, Monroe, Louisiana. When, in the first hours, they had difficulty breathing, Dr. Russell H. Bulloch went to the telephone and dialed long distance, area code 504, 837-BABY, the Ochsner pediatric department. He arranged to have a flying ambulance sent to pick up the infants.

Although Jones's own jet was faster, the Ochsner propeller plane is equipped with life-sustaining devices. Highly trained transport nurses and respiration therapists make the plane and ambulance trips. They are in constant contact by radio telephone with Ochsner pediatricians. Sometimes when birth difficulties are expected, the mothers-to-be are brought to Ochsner in order that the babies may be placed in the unit immediately. But it takes no longer than two hours to bring a patient from any part of Louisiana, and in its first six years of operation, no infant died while enroute to the hospital.

Waiting at the New Orleans Lakefront Airport on June 1, 1978, the morning the Jones twins arrived, was Jay P. Goldsmith, head of the pediatrics department and director of the neonatal intensive care unit. A native of Baltimore, Goldsmith had learned that his patients were the children of his favorite player on the Colts team. In the hospital the babies quickly responded to treatment, and two weeks later, the former Louisiana State University star and his wife, Danielle, flew them home to Ruston in the jet.

The happy ending is repeated in nearly 90 percent of the cases now treated in the facility, even though ten years ago fewer than half of the tiny premature children survived. The transport system went into action on July 5, 1976, when Goldsmith became head of pediatrics. On the following day the first delivery of a patient by plane was made. He was Eric Haik, three-pound premature child born at the Dauterive Hospital in New Iberia, Louisiana. Eric's father, State Representative Theodore M. Haik, Jr., later sponsored legislation creating the Louisiana Perinatal Commission. The chairman is Terry D. King, Goldsmith's predecessor at Ochsner. Since the commission came into being the newborn death rate in the state has been reduced from eighteen per thousand births to thirteen.

In the 1980s Ochsner continues the work the founders planned for it—care of the difficult cases and the most advanced care possible. Ochsner develops the new techniques that others will use and also employs the techniques others have devised just as soon as they can be safely performed.

Dr. Jefferson J. Kaye was getting ready to begin a busy day's schedule on March 16, 1981, when he had a call from the emergency room. He hurried downstairs to find an ironworker whose left hand had been severed at the wrist a few minutes earlier by a metal shear in a plant in nearby Harahan. The orthopedic surgeon dispatched a Jefferson Parish sheriff's deputy to the plant to retrieve the hand. Somebody on the scene had had the presence of mind to put the hand into ice, and it was in good shape when it was delivered to Kaye.

The patient, John S. Atchley, was moved to the surgical area in a room equipped for microsurgery, and Kaye prepared to reattach the hand. For ten and a half hours he worked at reconnecting arteries, veins, nerves, tendons, bone, and skin.

"When I woke up in the recovery room," Atchley related, "I looked at it and couldn't believe I had my hand back on. The fingers moved—right then, immediately! It was like waking up from a bad dream."

After weeks of therapy Atchley underwent a second operation to deal with scarring of nerves and tendons, and a year after the accident his hand functioned at 40 percent of normal. If it seemed a miracle to the ironworker, it was a miracle that represented the skill and research of an entire medical community focused in the dextrous hands of an Ochsner surgeon. Such miracles are the goal of Ochsner's founders, and they happen every day.

CHAPTER TEN

The Jefferson Highway Campus

On a clear, hot Saturday, June 12, 1954, staff doctors loaded seventy-two of the patients at Splinter Village into their personal automobiles and drove two miles along the Jefferson Highway to the new Ochsner Foundation Hospital. Sixty-two other more seriously ill persons were transported in ambulances. It was a journey out of the past into the gleaming future. From the barrackslike surroundings of the old wards, the 134 men, women, and children were transferred to a 250-bed facility that incorporated the advances of modern hospital architecture. The rooms even had doors, offering the luxury of privacy to the patients who had grown to expect the cubicles and the endless bustle of the frame buildings of Camp Plauché. It took some getting used to, and for a while nurses heard complaints about the isolation from ward mates.

Ochsner had found a permanent home. But it was only the beginning, a first step in the development of the complex that in three decades would cover 28.8 riverside acres. In the over thirty years since the first piling was driven for the new hospital in 1952, there has been no interval of more than a few months when the builders have not been busy on expansion projects and the planners on the blueprints for more facilities.

The scene that greeted the first patients bore little resemblance to the cluster of blond brick and glass structures that came to dominate the East Jefferson riverbank. In the weedpatch where the ponies of the riding academy had been stabled stood two modest newly completed buildings and a third structure on which workmen were putting the finishing touches. The five-story hospital was the centerpiece. It had cost $5,388,113, including the public donations netted from the area-wide drive, $1,325,000 of Hill-Burton funds appropriated by the federal government for new medical centers, and a mortgage loan from the Pan-American Life Insurance Company. To the west of the hospital was the two-story structure intended to provide a home for nurses. Constructed with a $354,985 contribution from the Libby-Dufour Foundation, it has always borne the name Libby-Dufour Building. It had barely been completed in time for the hospital opening. On the eastern edge of the tract Brent House hotel—named, of course, in honor of Theodore Brent—was several months from being ready for occupancy. The eighty-one-room facility would cost $764,553, of which $400,000 came from a mortgage loan from Pan-American and $300,000 was lent to the foundation by the Orleans Service Corporation, the association made up of staff doctors and employees that would operate the hotel. Until Brent House was ready for business toward the end of 1954, the foundation leased the Libby-Dufour Building to the Orleans Service Corporation to provide hotel accommodations for patients and their families. The nurses were housed in a motel on Airline Highway until the Libby-Dufour Building was vacated.

In the area near the unfinished Brent House on a site that became part of the paved employee parking lot was a trailer park, which produced a small income to the foundation for several years to come. Next door to Brent House was the lumberyard of the Southport Lumber Company, where a fire would later break out that would threaten the hospital complex. At 11:30 P.M. on October 5, 1968, the fire drove guests out of the hotel. The heat from the blaze was so intense that windows on the near side of the building were melted. Doctors hurried to the scene and stood by ready to evacuate patients from the hospital if necessary, as the flames lit up the night, but the fire was brought under control without further incident.

On moving day, 1954, a basic problem remained unsolved. The clinic was still housed in the building at Prytania and Aline streets and in nearby residential-type structures. True, the new hospital was two miles closer than Splinter Village had been, but a three-mile drive over city streets still separated the two activities. The staff was losing valuable hours in transit and patients were inconvenienced. The shuttle bus

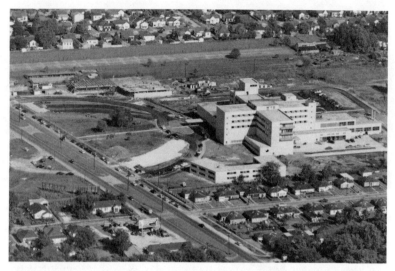

Aerial view of the new hospital as it looked on moving day, 1954
John L. Herrmann, FRPS

system devised to deliver patients and records was expensive and inefficient. The situation was exacerbated by insufficient space to accommodate the growing volume of clinic patients who sought treatment after
the lull of 1950–1951. Eventually, the foundation would have to find a
source for financing a clinic building alongside the hospital, as well as
for providing all of the facilities needed on the campus for handling
Ochsner's mushrooming activities. The story of how the Jefferson
Highway center was developed begins with the founders, especially
Guy A. Caldwell, and with trustees Richard W. Freeman and J. Blanc
Monroe, and it continues through the second generation, notably
Merrill Hines, and the third generation, principally Frank A. Riddick,
Jr., and George H. Porter III. Only Freeman was involved every step of
the lengthy way.

Richard Freeman became as influential in the affairs of the foundation in the 1960s and afterward as J. Blanc Monroe had been in the
earlier years. He was attracted to the institutions because of his admiration for the zeal of the founders, especially Alton Ochsner, and once
he was involved, he made the hospital and the research and education

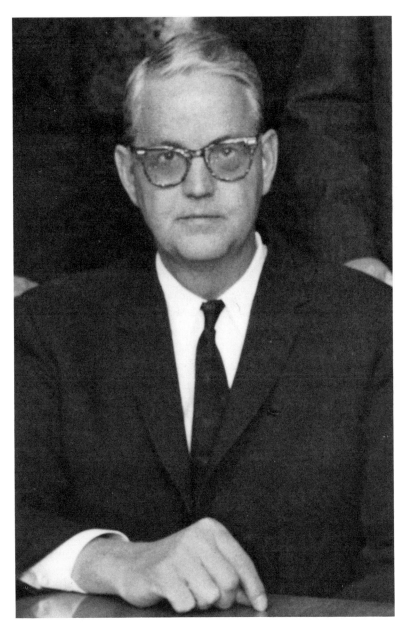

Richard W. Freeman

programs his principal civic interests. He served Delta Air Lines as chairman of the board and later as chairman of the finance committee, and he brought to the Ochsner councils the same acumen in business and financial matters that helped Delta progress from a crop-dusting service to one of the world's principal carriers. He was chairman of the Louisiana Coca-Cola Bottling Company, a business founded by his father, A. B. Freeman, and he was also director of New Orleans Public Service and Middle South Utilities. No other New Orleans executive of Freeman's active era was more successful or respected.

Richard Freeman inherited a sense of community responsibility and philanthropy. His posts included the presidencies of the Community Chest and International House. As a graduate of the Tulane School of Business Administration, Freeman served on the university's board of administrators and worked for the benefit of his alma mater with an energy second only to that he exerted on behalf of Ochsner. In the 1960s Freeman had a foot in each camp as officials of Ochsner and the Tulane medical school debated the idea of merging. Later he recalled that he and Darwin S. Fenner, president of the Tulane board, had been concerned over the cooling of relationships between Ochsner doctors and the medical school faculty and had encouraged a thaw. He explained that he and Fenner had no thought of a union, and he was surprised when discussions took such a turn.

Freeman ruled as Rex, King of Carnival, in 1959; received Tulane's Outstanding Alumnus Award in 1975; and won the *Times-Picayune* Loving Cup for civic service in 1977. His involvement with the Ochsner Institutions covers the entire period of the building of the present campus.

A year and a half before the hospital was completed the partners were exploring the possibility of constructing a building for the clinic on the grounds. On January 13, 1953, Ellerbe and Company estimated the cost of a facility to provide offices for seventy-five or eighty physicians at $1,750,000. Building No. 4, as it was referred to in discussions and correspondence, was beyond the means of the foundation at the time, even though the need was becoming more and more urgent. Caldwell looked over the property in the neighborhood of the old clinic in the hope of finding temporary space that might allow expansion of the clinic staff without waiting for a building on Jefferson Highway. The only suitable prospect was the Sunday school building of the First Baptist Church, at Delachaise and St. Charles Avenue. Caldwell said the building could be remodeled to provide offices for sixty or seventy doctors. He suggested it would permit the establishment of such departments as ophthalmology, dermatology, oral surgery, and plastic surgery and would allow the size of the internal medicine staff to double. He estimated that such an expansion would cost $600,000 to $700,000 a year but might produce additional revenue of as much as $1 million. On July 27, 1954, the clinic board of administrators adopted a resolution asking the trustees of the foundation to acquire the property for lease to the clinic. However, the church declined to lease the building and set a selling price of $250,000, although the real estate expert Stanley M. Lemarie rated the value at only $175,000. Later, the trustees (five of the seven of whom were members of the clinic board of administrators) decided that it would be impractical to spend money on a stopgap solution.

Monroe, Freeman, and the founders were discussing the possibility of constructing a small cheap building on the hospital grounds to provide offices for some of the clinic doctors when Rawley M. Penick suggested the idea that resulted in the pacesetting project for all of the expansion that has occurred at the Ochsner center. In the summer of 1955, he proposed that two floors be added to Brent House, so designed that the space could be used for clinic offices for a while and then converted to hotel rooms. Monroe concluded a readjustment of the foundation's mortgage with the Pan-American Life Insurance Company that provided $500,000, and the two floors were begun. The cost, in all, was $512,805. In the spring of 1957 the Brent House Division of the Ochsner Clinic was opened. Alton Ochsner moved into the area, along with the department of general surgery, neurosurgery, orthopedic surgery, neurology, psychiatry, pediatrics, allergy, and endocrinology.

The first new structure added to the compound after its opening was the facility later named the Richard W. Freeman Research Institute, which was completed in May, 1959. The building contains the research laboratories and experimental animal colonies. It was constructed at a cost of $747,505, of which the National Institutes of Health contributed $200,000 and the Libby-Dufour Foundation $50,000.

By 1956 the 250 beds of the hospital could no longer fill the needs of the growing clinic staff, and the Ochsner founders had evidence to support a concept that they had known in theory since the early days. In order for the institutions to prosper, there had to be a balance among the components. If a significant number of beds were to be added to the hospital, the clinic staff would have to be enlarged in order to provide patients to fill them. If the clinic hired additional doctors, the hospital's capacity would have to be increased to handle their referrals. If clinic and hospital grew, then the Brent House hotel needed more rooms for the patients and their families who flocked in from out of town and from Latin America. If the hospital became bigger, then for the sake of efficiency the graduate training program would have to supply more interns and residents as house staff. Ever since the present campus was opened, balance has been a keynote of planning. One result has been an absence of pressure on clinic doctors to fill empty hospital beds, no temptation to admit patients for unneeded procedures because of gaping vacancies.

Two floors, the sixth and seventh, were added to the hospital in a project that was completed in October, 1960. The expansion provided a total of 362 beds and narrowed the gap in size between Ochsner and the largest of the private New Orleans hospitals, Touro Infirmary and Southern Baptist. Caldwell took the initiative in negotiating a grant of Hill-Burton funds from the Louisiana State Hospital Board and managed to obtain $462,407 toward the total cost of $1,850,000. The rest of the money needed was raised in an unpublicized campaign for donations from citizens who had shown previous interest in Ochsner.

Ten years of effort brought reward on March 18, 1963, with the opening of the new six-story clinic building adjacent to the hospital. Its construction was not by any means the most expensive project the foundation undertook in the development of the campus, but none of the other programs was as difficult to finance. Caldwell, Freeman, and Monroe spent endless hours in planning and negotiations before a contract of $3,384,000 for constructing a six-story building finally was awarded on May 25, 1961. The purchase of equipment brought the total to $4 million. The problem was that the foundation's only source of cash for a down payment would be from the sale of the old clinic properties—which eventually realized only $692,000. Since a mortgage would have to be paid off with rentals from the clinic, the amount would be limited by the partnership's ability to pay. The revenue brought in by a staff restricted by the old facilities would not support even a scaled-down new building, but consultants reported that the volume of income at clinics that expanded their offices had without exception increased from 15 to 25 percent. Administrator Edgar J. Saux predicted that the revenue of the clinic would rise to $5 million in the first full year of operation on the campus. This amount would allow the clinic to pay a rental in line with the going rate for medical space and would permit the foundation to borrow for a building.

Meanwhile, the Texas oil tycoon Clint Murchison set his lieutenants to the task of trying to arrange financing for a clinic building. Finally, Murchison and his allies devised a plan under which they would purchase the Charles Town horse-racing track in West Virginia and, once it was operating at a profit, donate it to the foundation. Murchison's idea was that the track would provide a continuing source of income for the Ochsner Institutions. Two or three members of the foundation board of governors expressed reluctance over having the institutions operate a track at which pari-mutuel gambling was conducted. Then Murchison's attorney telephoned to relay an offer from outside interests to buy Charles Town for a net to the foundation of $400,000. Caldwell tried in vain to reach Murchison himself by telephone before the meeting of the trustees. At that meeting, Ochsner spoke strongly in favor of accepting the offer, and the board voted to do so. Apparently, the sale miffed Murchison, who knew nothing of his attorney's offer, but the board's decision was undoubtedly a wise one. Certainly the profit from the sale was a generous gift, and Murchison's name is listed with those of Sid W. Richardson, Vernon Neuhaus, Perry R. Bass, Don Harrington, Billy G. Byers, and Wofford Cain on a plaque in the lobby. These were the main donors, "whose help made this building possible."

Unusual as the gift of a racetrack may sound, it was not the only unorthodox donation made over the years. Gifts have included oil royalties and real estate, as well as cash, stocks, and bonds. In 1952 Theodore Brent made a gift of the Coast Transportation Company, then in

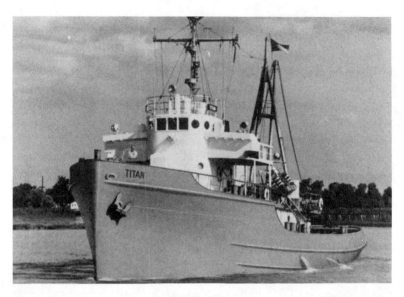

The tugboat *Titan*

liquidation, which was valued at $400,000. Among the assets acquired was a seagoing tugboat, the *Titan*, which was leased to a barge line. After the foundation became defendant in damage suits growing out of collisions in which the *Titan* was involved, however, the tug was sold in 1954 for $175,000.

With the cash from the sale of the Prytania Street properties and the racetrack and a mortgage loan from the Pan-American Life Insurance Company, the clinic building was constructed and all of the Ochsner activities finally brought together on one campus twenty-one years after the Tulane professors began their group practice. The doctors abandoned the Physicians and Surgeons Building in which they had begun their practice together, but not without misgivings. Francis Le-Jeune worried about how the children he treated in his ear, nose, and throat practice would make their way to the suburban Jefferson Parish site. But he and the others need not have worried; the trustees' optimism was amply justified. In the first full year after the move, clinic revenues exceeded Saux's $5 million forecast, and the billings of Le-Jeune's department were a third greater than before.

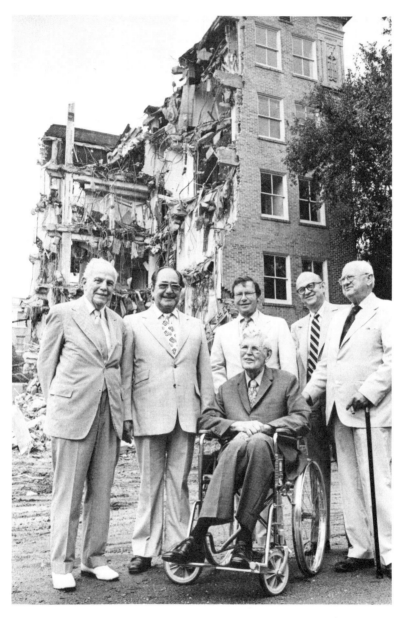

At the demolition of the old clinic building. *Left to right*: Alton Ochsner, Edgar Saux, Frank Riddick, Merrill Hines, Curtis Tyrone, and Guy Caldwell (in wheelchair)

The clinic building might well have borne Caldwell's name, for it was the last addition to the campus for which he and other founders were, along with Freeman, the active planners. By the time the next project was begun, Caldwell had turned over the medical directorship and membership on the board of trustees to Merrill Hines, and the second generation had taken over.

Merrill Hines originated the idea for a Rawley M. Penick Memorial Pavilion, the next building to be completed. The pavilion was named for one of the second-generation partners. Penick began working at the clinic on September 1, 1942, and he remained an Ochsner doctor until his death on February 21, 1963. After obtaining his medical degree in 1924, he remained at Johns Hopkins for seven years of postgraduate training before coming to New Orleans as an instructor at Tulane. Later, he served for twelve years as professor of clinical surgery at Tulane after a stint as professor of surgery at Louisiana State University. Rawley Penick was largely responsible for the development of the Tumor Registry at Charity Hospital, and so it is appropriate that the building that bears his name houses Ochsner's nuclear medicine and radiation therapy departments. The two-story structure also provided for expansion of the busy emergency room. It was completed in the summer of 1967 at a cost of $1,546,614, of which $250,000 was provided by a Hill-Burton grant. Memorial donations from Penick's friends and foundation reserves paid the difference.

Two years after the opening of the Penick Pavilion, the foundation financed a thirty-six-room addition to Brent House, completed at a cost of $500,000. Then, having tested its management talents with these two projects, the second generation, abetted by Freeman, ventured into a more ambitious program by launching a drive for funds in 1968. The last of the founders had retired from the board of trustees, and Freeman and Hines were playing their Mr. Outside and Mr. Inside parts in earnest.

The "Pursuit of Excellence" campaign brought in public donations to finance a $3,784,046 expansion of hospital facilities. Campaign workers, eager to capitalize on his fame, named Alton Ochsner honorary chairman of the campaign organization. He never missed a fundraising assignment, but this was essentially a new-breed activity. Richard Freeman and Morrell F. Trimble were general cochairmen. The

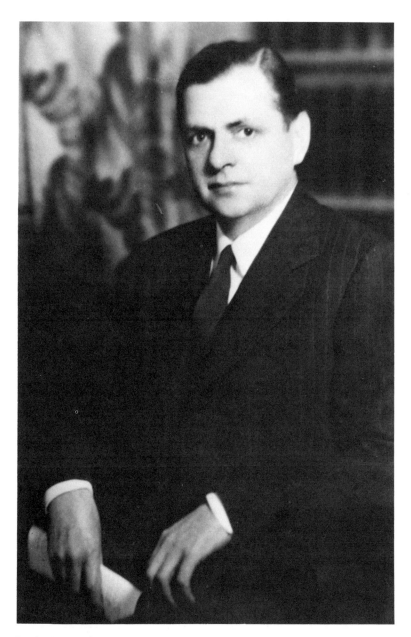

Rawley M. Penick, Jr.

successful campaign financed two-story additions to the side and front of the hospital building and new stories atop low-rise sections of the structure. The space between the tower of the hospital and clinic was filled in with new offices. New operating rooms were added, along with a new intensive care unit, enlarged administrative areas, and a ground-floor auditorium that bears the name of Blanc Monroe. The work, begun in 1971 and completed the following year, set the stage for a program in the 1974–1979 period that dwarfed anything that had been done on the campus before.

By the time the "Pursuit of Excellence" improvements were completed, the clinic partnership agreement of 1971 had presaged the eventual passage of control of the institutions from the second generation to the third. Coincidentally, Ochsner was coming to a crossroads. A growing influx of patients was straining the capacity of the facilities and taxing the capability of the existing clinic medical staff to serve the demands on it. New and expanding hospitals by then were competing for patients, and the decision of the Tulane University School of Medicine to establish a faculty practice in a Tulane Medical Center meant that for the first time a rival clinic approaching the size of Ochsner would be in business in New Orleans. Ochsner would either have to turn away patients (to the benefit of competing doctors and hospitals) or arrange to have a large enough staff and a sufficient number of beds to accommodate everybody who sought medical care. Neither the second generation nor the third had any intention of allowing Ochsner to yield its preeminence.

Along with the problem came opportunity. In 1968 the state legislature created the Health Education Authority of Louisiana, known as HEAL, which was charged with implementing a master plan for the development of a medical complex. The primary institutions involved would be Charity Hospital of Lousiana in New Orleans, the medical center of the Louisiana State University, and the medical center of the Tulane School of Medicine. Other organizations in the vicinity of the Charity Hospital could come into HEAL as participating institutions. Later, when Richard Freeman and the trustees saw the advantages offered to participating institutions, HEAL officials went to the legislature and had the eligibility broadened to include organizations within a ten-mile radius of Charity Hospital. This enabled Ochsner to be included.

HEAL opened up a source of financing beyond the dreams of the Ochsner trustees who had spent so many years in public solicitation and negotiating with governmental agencies to scrape together the total of not quite $20 million needed to bring the campus to the stage of development that it had reached after the "Pursuit of Excellence." HEAL's charter allowed the authority to issue tax-free revenue bonds on behalf of participating institutions. The bonded debt could be paid out of revenues, and the so-called municipal bond tax exemption meant that an issue could be sold at favorable interest rates virtually guaranteed to attract buyers without burdening the borrower with the percentages charged for private corporation debt. Caldwell, who had always strenuously objected to having clinic outpatients pay higher fees in order to support a hospital that they were not entering, must have been pleased with the concept of having the users pay for the improvement of the facilities that they enjoyed.

The Ochsner planners began mapping out a program of a magnitude that in China could have been called a Great Leap Forward. They proposed to change the face of the campus at a cost, including financing, of $61,571,000. Construction alone, without taking into account new equipment, would run to $45,401,000—more than double the total outlay for all of the existing buildings.

For the first time, the third generation of staff physicians joined the second generation in the planning. The leader from the younger staff was Frank A. Riddick, Jr., associate medical director and heir apparent to Merrill Hines, who would have to step aside in 1975 because of his age. Riddick helped Hines carry the ball in scrimmages that had to be won before the project could be started.

Ochsner received a setback when the staff of the New Orleans Area Health Planning Council recommended that the project be scaled down before receiving the required approval of the council. The council said New Orleans was already well supplied with physicians and did not need the added members contemplated for the clinic. Figures were cited to show that New Orleans had 2.27 physicians per thousand of population, while Indianapolis had 1.75, Portland 2.01,

Tampa–St. Petersburg 1.45, Atlanta 1.78, and Houston 1.64. The council report also said that Ochsner's need for an additional 380 employees would seriously drain the critically small pool of registered nurses. Hines and Riddick appeared before the project review committee of the council to point out that increasing numbers of patients were seeking care at Ochsner. Riddick added that only fifty-seven of the additional employees needed would be nurses. He also argued that the Ochsner Medical Center "functions as a referral medical facility with a national and international reputation for its quality, is regional in nature consisently drawing 50% to 60% of its patients from outside this planning area." The council was persuaded, and the plan approved.

This skirmish was only a warm-up for the decisive battle that the leadership fought out at two meetings of the clinic partnership in the fall of 1974. Two disclosures had raised questions among the partners. One was that the rent paid by the clinic to the foundation would be increased from $341,385 per year to $1,568,208 once the clinic building was enlarged. The other was that the radiology department and the pathology laboratories would have to become operations of the foundation rather than the clinic, with a potential loss of income to the partnership. The reason for the change was an Internal Revenue Service regulation that disallows the issuance of tax-free bonds if more than 25 percent of the proceeds are used to finance any undertaking which is not itself tax-exempt. The foundation is tax-exempt, but the clinic is not. Hines, Freeman, and Riddick explained that the costs of the clinic expansion could not be held within the 25 percent limit if essential improvements were made in radiology and pathology while they remained clinic activities, but the work could be done if they were part of the foundation. Hines, Freeman, and Riddick also noted that, in addition to paying rent, the clinic had donated $4,127,100 to the foundation in the period beginning in 1965. Thus, the new rent would not actually represent much increase in the payments of clinic to foundation. These arguments persuaded the partners, who voted unanimously to support the expansion. But after its completion, the clinic suspended its annual contributions to the foundation. Subsequently, doctors donated to the foundation only on an individual basis.

In 1975 HEAL issued bonds for the Ochsner's project in the amount of $56,200,000 at an average interest rate of 8.54 percent. The last of

the bonds are payable in the year 2005. In carrying out the legal requirements, the foundation leased the campus to HEAL, which then
subleased the property back to the foundation. The foundation put
$3 million of its own capital into the expansion, and added $2,371,000
that was received in interest on the bond money while construction
was in progress.

The bonds that made the project possible bear the name of a second-
generation Ochsner official. When a committee went to the New York
office of the underwriter to carry out the signing formalities, L. R. Jordan, president of the Alton Ochsner Medical Foundation, sat down at
a table and prepared to affix his signature. An immediate objection
came from Merrill Hines. "I am chairman of the board of trustees," he
said. "I am the senior official of the Ochsner Foundation, and I am the
one who should sign these bonds." Richard Freeman agreed, and Jordan gave way.

The Jefferson Highway complex reached skyward in the vast building program that was completed in 1978. Four stories were added to
the hospital and five to the clinic to create a massive structure that ap-
pears to be a single eleven-story building, by now the most prominent
landmark on the East Bank of the Mississippi River between Audubon
Park and the Huey P. Long Bridge. The hospital capacity was increased
by 131 beds. In all, the hospital expansion cost $29,257,000 in con-
struction costs alone. The clinic enlargement provided accommodations for 59 additional doctors, or a total staff of 140, at a cost of
$13,831,000.

The expansion was horizontal as well as vertical, with three new
structures being added to the group of buildings. A strip of land on the
east side of the Riding Academy site was leased for construction of a
six-story parking garage, providing space for 1,470 automobiles,
which was built at a cost of $6,968,000. On the Jefferson Highway
side, six stories were added to Brent House. The 102 new rooms
brought the total number of rooms to 260, and the construction cost
was $3,624,000. Behind the hospital, the foundation built a two-story
materials management building for the handling and storage of supplies. The cost of $4,100,000 was included in the total for the hospital
expansion.

As prodigious as it was, the great leap of the middle 1970s carried the institutions only into the summer of 1982, when new projects were underway. These were the first building expansions engineered solely by the third generation, now holding down the management posts, with Porter as president of the foundation and Riddick as medical director of the clinic.

Porter had a telephone call one day in 1980 from William G. Geary, head of the obstetrical-gynecological department. He asked Porter and J. Thomas Lewis, chairman of the board of trustees, to meet him that afternoon in the obstetrical area of the hospital. Geary led a tour through the facilities, pointing out that the rooms lacked natural light and, although they were thoroughly modern, offered little appeal to happy new mothers. Geary proposed that a new floor be built above the hospital laboratories to house a bright new obstetrical unit that would win the admiration of patients. Ironically, only eight years earlier Lewis had been a member of a committee appointed to consider abandonment of the hospital's obstetrical service, which was not paying its way. The committee had voted unanimously to continue the unit, and it eventually became overcrowded. Porter and Lewis liked Geary's ideas, put in-house architects to work, and won trustee approval for a $3.7 million project. The improvements include the obstetrics unit, a nursery for newborns, and renovation of the cardiology area to provide more private rooms for patients who have heart surgery.

An increasing flow of Latin American patients necessitated the addition of a six-story wing to Brent House, construction that brought the total number of rooms to 374. Two shelled-in floors will allow future expansion, and if even more new rooms are ever needed, the foundation will support an eleven-story building. The project was the first to be carried out after the Alton Ochsner Medical Foundation acquired Brent House on November 1, 1979, from the Orleans Service Corporation. The hotel is now operated by the Brent House Corporation, a subsidiary of the foundation.

In the lobby of the hospital hang the portraits of six surgeons and one layman—seven of the nine men who made the greatest contributions to the growth of the institutions. On the west wall, side by side, are oils of the five founders painted by Clay Parker, who started the collection in 1954 by donating his rendition of Alton Ochsner. The clinic staff then commissioned the artist to paint the portraits of Guy

A. Caldwell, Francis E. LeJeune, Edgar Burns, and Curtis H. Tyrone. On the south wall are paintings of Merrill O. Hines, also executed by Parker and hung in 1975, and of Richard Freeman, painted by Everett Raymond Kinstler and hung in 1982. Down the corridor a few steps away is the entrance to Monroe Hall, named in honor of J. Blanc Monroe, the attorney and trustee who shaped the clinic and foundation. In the hall is displayed a painting of Monroe, together with Theodore Brent. The two were the first laymen trustees of the foundation, and Brent was the first major benefactor.

CHAPTER ELEVEN

A Bright Heritage and Sorrow

A call for Doctor Ochsner over the paging system of the Ochsner Foundation Hospital could make the lights start flashing on the telephone switchboard. Over the years, many Ochsners have served the facility that bears Alton Ochsner's name. Not only the founder himself but also his three sons, a daughter-in-law, a granddaughter, and two cousins have at various times been on the professional staff.

The first of Alton Ochsner's kin to join the staff, on August 15, 1946, was his cousin Albert John Ochsner, grandson of A. J. Ochsner, the eminent Chicago surgeon who was Alton's mentor. Albert John Ochsner was an anesthesiologist on the Ochsner staff until April 1, 1952, when he resigned to enter practice at Alexandria, Louisiana. His brother, Seymour F. Ochsner, one of the nation's leading radiologists, has been connected with the institutions since July 1, 1953. He has headed the departments of radiology and radiation therapy and has served as assistant medical director.

The first of Alton Ochsner's three sons to join his father professionally was Alton, Jr., a general surgeon, who became affiliated on January 1, 1958. He left on October 30, 1968, and practices independently in the New Orleans area. His daughter Coller began a residency in dermatology on July 1, 1980.

John Lockwood Ochsner, Alton's second son, was recruited on January 16, 1961, and has headed the department of surgery since 1966. Alton Ochsner's eyes used to light up whenever he talked about his son John. "He's the best surgeon I ever saw," the patriarch would say, and his offspring's accomplishments made it clear that there was more than

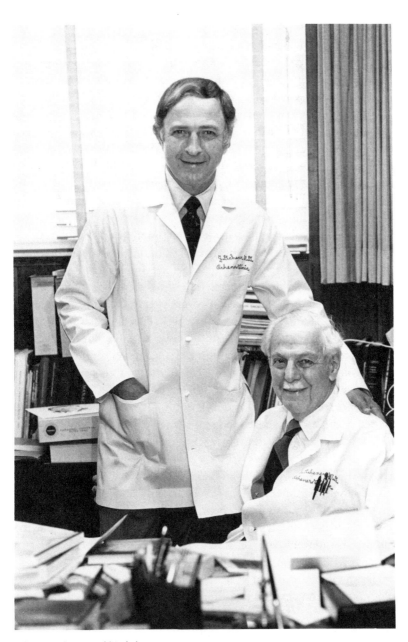

John L. Ochsner and his father

paternal pride in this judgment. The younger Ochsner was associated with surgeons Michael E. DeBakey and Denton Cooley in Houston in 1960 when the clinic was looking around for a candidate to replace Alton as head of surgery when he retired. Merrill O. Hines accompanied the elder Ochsner to Houston for a discussion with John. The New Orleanians had dinner with DeBakey and told him the purpose of their visit. "How much will you pay him?" DeBakey asked. "Sixteen thousand," Hines replied. "I'll offer him twice that to stay here," De-Bakey said, "but if he wants to go I won't stand in the way." Hines made his pitch, and young Ochsner reluctantly gave up an opportunity for a brilliant career as an associate of DeBakey. "After all, my name is over the door," he explains.

John Ochsner already had attracted attention as a pediatric surgeon and was doing pioneer investigative work in the development of techniques for bypass surgery. He and Noel L. Mills collaborated to give the clinic a head start in the perfection of the bypass procedure that is now performed thousands of times every year in hospitals throughout the country. Nearing the peak of his active years, Ochsner has won international recognition as a worthy successor to a famous father. His election to office in international surgical societies reflects his eminence.

A restless innovator, Ochsner has found time to contribute to advances in other areas as well as in bypass surgery. He performed the only heart transplant carried out in Louisiana; he was the first in the United States to transpose the great vessels of a heart; he installed a pacemaker in the body of the youngest patient of record.

In 1966 he restored the circulation of blood to the crippled foot of a sixty-five-year-old woman by making a graft from a vein in her leg and stretching it from knee to ankle, bypassing an occluded tibial artery. A gangrenous toe had to be removed, but the patient was able to walk again. Ochsner and his colleague Paul T. DeCamp in 1966 pioneered the use of cadaver veins for grafts to save the feet and lower legs of patients with clogged arteries.

He was joined the next year by James F. Arens, chief of anesthesiology, and Glenn Gee, a therapist, in devising an apparatus that allows long-term respiratory assistance without damage to the trachea. In positive-pressure ventilation, air is forced into the lungs through a tube placed in the trachea either through the nose or through an incision in the throat. The tube includes a cuff, which must fit tightly against the wall of the trachea when the patient is inhaling. The pressure of the cuff causes sores in about half of the patients. The Ochsner-Arens-Gee equipment is designed to inflate the cuff during the inhalations and to deflate it during the exhalations. The intermittent deflation relieves the pressure and enables patients to receive inhalation therapy for weeks at a time without complications.

In 1972 Ochsner, Noel Mills, George L. Leonard, and Noel Lawson reported a method of reducing postoperative complications of open-heart surgery by using a patient's own blood for transfusions. The detrimental effects of the heart-lung machine on blood had long been recognized, but transfusions of donor blood put the patient at risk of contracting hepatitis or other infections. Clinic doctors began drawing out 20 percent of a patient's blood just before the operation and storing it. The volume is replaced with a lactate solution. After the open-heart surgery, which necessitates employment of the heart-lung pump; the stored blood is returned to the veins, rejuvenating the damaged blood. The Ochsner team demonstrated that patients who received their own blood were spared the risk of infection and had fewer problems with postoperative bleeding.

But not all operations are successful. John Ochsner's hopes of emulating the success of his father in separating the Mouton twins proved impossible of fulfillment in late 1982. Twin girls, joined at the chest and upper abdomen, were born on Christmas Day to an eighteen-year-old mother, delivered by Caesarean section performed by John B. Holland. One heart supplied blood to both of the premature babies, and the twin who was deprived of a heart also lacked a liver. In a four-hour operation Ochsner and pediatric surgeon Robert M. Arensman, along with plastic surgeon John M. Finley, freed the complete girl from her lesser sister. The survivor left the operating table in stable condition but unexpectedly died two hours later. An autopsy revealed that the heart was defective, and Ochsner had no way of knowing whether he could have effected repairs if the baby had lived long enough for the attempt to be made.

On September 25, 1961, Alton Ochsner's youngest son came onto the staff. Mims Gage Ochsner was named for his father's closest friend, Idys Mims Gage, a surgeon who, as an early member of the clinic staff,

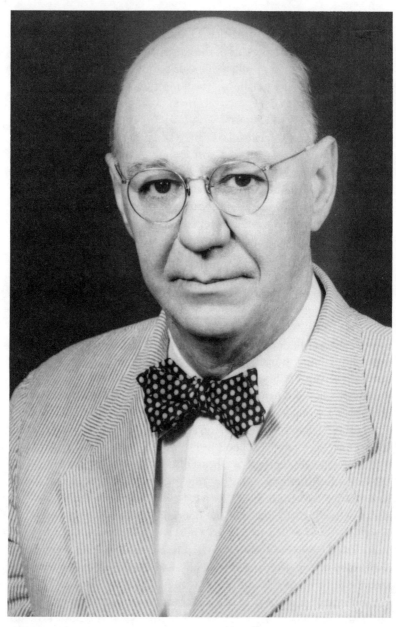

Idys Mims Gage

added luster to its name. As a senior member of the surgical faculty at Tulane, Gage gave Alton Ochsner warm support during his early years as chairman of the department when the newcomer was under fire from rivals who had hoped to occupy the chair themselves. Ochsner never forgot Gage's loyalty. He enlisted him as a consultant in surgery for the opening of the clinic. A medical officer during World War II, Gage organized the Tulane General Hospital Unit in 1942 and served with the army for three years, leaving with the rank of colonel and winning a Legion of Merit ribbon. He rejoined the clinic staff full time on November 1, 1945, and was active until his death on December 12, 1957. Mims Gage is remembered not only for his skill with a scalpel but also for his almost mystical talent for diagnosis. His portrait in army uniform hangs in the Ochsner medical library, to which he donated his extensive collection of professional volumes.

His Ochsner namesake has been associate head of the department of urology since 1970. Mims Gage Ochsner's wife, Rise Delmar Ochsner, joined the department of ophthalmology on August 1, 1976.

The hospital on the Jefferson Highway to which Alton Ochsner gave his name turned into a house of sorrow for the surgeon. Within a year of the opening of the facility came the first personal tragedy, the death on May 4, 1955, of 2½-year-old Edgar Allen Davis, Jr., Ochsner's first grandson. The little boy was one of the children who succumbed to poliomyelitis after being inoculated with the Salk vaccine in the early days of the program that by now has almost wiped out the threat of the crippling disease. The deaths were blamed on the inadvertent inclusion of live polio viruses among the killed viruses in the injections that provided immunity to millions of children. Ochsner's grief was compounded on May 19, when Daniel Trigg, one of the resident physicians who treated young Davis, was hospitalized with polio. Although Trigg's exposure through the patient was total—he may even have given the child mouth-to-mouth resuscitation—it was not clear whether he contracted the disease in this way. He also had been exposed when his own young son became ill after receiving the vaccine. His child recovered. Although confined to a wheelchair, Trigg returned to the hospital and began residency training in pathology, a specialty that he could practice in the laboratory despite his physical handicap.

Ochsner was further saddened by a controversial aftermath to his grandson's death. His daughter Isabel "Sis" Ochsner Davis and her husband, Allen Davis, Sr., public affairs director for the Ochsner Institutions, filed suit against Cutter Laboratories, makers of the vaccine. A number of clinic doctors, led by Dean Echols, objected on the grounds that Cutter was making a major contribution to medicine in helping to conquer polio and should not be penalized for an unfortunate accident. Alton Ochsner, Jr., then a member of the general surgery staff, spoke in defense of the Davises' action, but they later withdrew the suit.

The shadows in the hospital corridors grew even darker for Alton Ochsner, Sr., on April 4, 1968, when his wife for more than forty years, Isabel Lockwood Ochsner, died. Isabel Ochsner had been in the facility on and off for six months for treatment of adenocarcinoma of the lung, which developed in a scar caused by a bout with pneumonia ten years earlier. It was, without question, the saddest day in Ochsner's life.

Thirteen years later the eighty-five-year-old Ochsner bought airline tickets and arranged to leave on September 4, 1981, with his second wife, Jane Kellogg Ochsner, for Greece, where he was scheduled to be honored at a surgical society convention in Athens. His son John, an officer in the association, was already in Athens for the convention. On September 1 the elder Ochsner complained of not feeling well and went to see a cardiologist, C. Lynn Skelton. Skelton told him to go home and rest and advised him to cancel the trip. As he was leaving his office, Ochsner stopped at the door and said to Gertrude Forshag, his private secretary for more than fifty years, "You know, it's a good thing John is in Greece. It would be too traumatic for him if he had to do a heart operation on me. But I've got a lot of faith in Noel Mills." Ochsner told her that he had an aortic stenosis, a blockage of the main artery at the point where it leaves the heart. Gertrude Forshag was shocked; Ochsner had kept the condition a secret from her since 1972, when a heart murmur indicative of the stenosis was discovered. Examinations in 1976 and 1978 had confirmed the condition.

On Friday, September 4, the day on which they had planned to leave for Greece, Jane Ochsner drove her husband to the hospital, where he was found to be seriously ill of congestive heart failure. He called Noel Mills into his room, and "clearly stated," said Mills, "that if things did

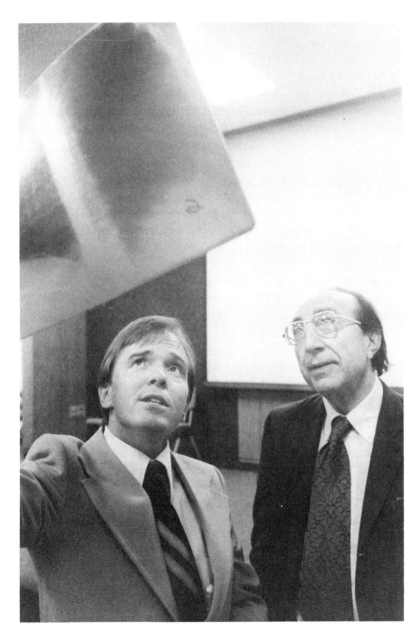

Noel Mills and Michael DeBakey

deteriorate he wanted me to take the bull by the horns and operate on him." By Sunday morning the patient's condition was worsening. He had apparently had a heart attack after entering the hospital. Cardiac catheterization confirmed calcification of the aortic valve and blockage of a coronary artery. Jane Ochsner consulted John in Greece and his two physician brothers, and all agreed that Mills should perform bypass surgery. Merrill Hines, watching the catheterization procedure, bent over Ochsner and told him surgery would be advisable. "Do what is necessary, Merrill," Ochsner responded.

And so, on Sunday, September 4, 1981, assisted by a team hastily recalled from Labor Day holidays, Mills performed on Alton Ochsner one of the open-heart procedures that he and John Ochsner had helped to perfect. He replaced the aortic valve with a synthetic substitute and bypassed one of the occluded heart vessels. The repaired heart functioned satisfactorily, but interstitial fibrosis of the lungs—thickening tissue that interfered with respiratory exchange of oxygen and carbon dioxide—developed. Only once in almost three weeks did physicians remove the tubes that helped Ochsner breathe. Within hours they had to return him to the support system. He died at 12:30 P.M. on September 24. In choosing to undergo surgery, Ochsner was true to the guiding philosophy of a long and celebrated career: Do something.

The two surviving founders watched on October 3, 1981, while hundreds of friends and admirers paid tribute to Ochsner at memorial services conducted in front of the hospital. Governor David Treen of Louisiana read a communication from President and Mrs. Ronald Reagan praising the surgeon.

The ninety-year-old Guy A. Caldwell looked on from a window on the eleventh floor of the hospital, where he was confined for his last illness. He died on November 1, 1981. Curtis H. Tyrone, eighty-three, had been injured in a fall. He was rolled in a wheelchair to a place in the audience. The end for the youngest of the five professors and the last remaining came on July 13, 1982.

CHAPTER TWELVE

The Dynamics of Leadership

Alone of the big six clinics, Ochsner is the creature of the doctor-partners on its staff. It has no organizational ties to the foundation, and the only laymen who sit in its councils are its own employees. The clinic makes no reports to the board of trustees of the foundation. In the other five clinics, trustee laymen have at least a token voice in affairs, although in practice the doctors run their own shows. All physicians on the staff of the Cleveland Clinic are salaried employees of the Cleveland Clinic Foundation, which is administered by a board of trustees composed of laymen and doctors. The trustees have delegated management responsibility to the board of governors, all physicians elected by the staff. The Lovelace Medical Foundation is a holding company that operates subsidiaries, including the medical practice. Authority rests with an executive committee made up of six laymen and five staff doctors, although a staff board of governors does the day-by-day medical supervision. The Lahey Clinic Foundation trustees, most of them laymen, have control over the LCF Foundation, the subsidiary that operates the clinic. At the Henry Ford Hospital, founded by Henry Ford, a mixed lay and professional board of trustees is responsible for the entire enterprise. The trustees appoint department chairmen and set their compensation. The Mayo Clinic Mayo Foundation Board of Trustees has full authority but leaves supervision over the practice of medicine to the board of governors, made up of the medical trustees.

At Ochsner, the doctors have managed to keep the control in their own hands despite changes in the organization of the institutions and at least one threat to their ascendancy. The interdependence of clinic and foundation was and is undeniable, but thanks to Blanc Monroe's unshakable conviction, the two remain separate. He and Richard W. Freeman were able, through force of personality and business acumen, to mold the foundation to fit their ideas. Had there ever been a showdown on the board of trustees, however, laymen would have been outvoted five to two.

When Ochsner appealed to the public for funds to build a hospital in the early 1950s, it was inevitable that those who had so generously donated their money would want a hand in running the hospital they had made possible. Raymond Rich, the fund raiser the doctors had hired, urged them to keep the most effective fund-raising civic leaders involved. If the men and women were enlisted for volunteer roles in hospital activities, he said, they would feel that Ochsner was respecting their advice as well as their donations. Rich suggested that the most active of the workers be added to the board of trustees of the foundation. To do this, it would be necessary to expand the board to a membership of fifty or sixty—too unwieldy, Rich conceded, to conduct business. But, he argued, this objection could be overcome by creating an executive committee with authority to make decisions. He was, it turned out, twenty years too early.

Trustees J. Blanc Monroe and Richard W. Freeman and the founders resisted the introduction of new faces on the tight-knit board but came up with a compromise that they felt would serve the purpose. They created a board of governors of the Ochsner Foundation Hospital. Members from the top strata of the New Orleans business, professional, and social communities were joined by several out-of-towners with impressive credentials. The list of those who were willing to become identified with the medical center reflected the public respect that Ochsner had won in the dozen years since the establishment of the clinic. At the first meeting, on June 15, 1954, insurance executive Gary Gillis was elected chairman. William O. Turner, president of the Louisiana Power and Light Company, became vice-chairman. Malcolm L. Monroe, J. Blanc's lawyer son, served as the first secretary. Other chairmen who presided over the governors in later years were Turner; A. Q. Peterson, cottonseed-oil magnate; and Joseph W. Montgomery, vice-president of the United Fruit Company.

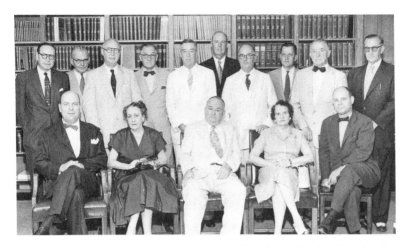

Part of the first Board of Governors of the Ochsner Foundation Hospital. *Seated, left to right*: Gary Gillis, Mrs. Laura Howard, Howell Crosby, Mrs. Russell Clark, Charles H. Murphy, Jr.; *standing*: Joseph Epstein, Parrish Fuller, A. Q. Petersen, Joseph W. Montgomery, Garner H. Tullis, Summerfield G. Roberts, Hollis Crosby, Malcolm Monroe, Edmund E. Richardson, and David Lide

On the first board, appointed by the trustees, were Howell Crosby and his brother Hollis, whose family has been the heaviest contributor to the Ochsner Institutions over the years. Other non–New Orleanians included Charles H. Murphy, Jr., of the Arkansas family that founded the Murphy Oil Company, and Parrish Fuller, a lumberman from Oakdale, Louisiana. William G. Helis, Jr., whose family financed and equipped the laboratories of the new hospital, was one of the New Orleans members. The three women on the original board were Mrs. Laura Howard, Mrs. Russell Clark, and Mrs. Wayne G. Borah, all of New Orleans. Mrs. Clark took the lead in arranging for the landscaping of the campus, with the help of John W. Murchison of Texas. She and her husband also provided the fountain, the centerpiece of the Ochsner grounds. Mrs. Howard was largely instrumental in obtaining the money for building the Libby-Dufour nurses' residence. After the building was opened, she felt the nurses should have a swimming pool and set about providing one. J. Blanc Monroe objected because he felt that raising funds for the project might interfere with a drive to finance an expansion of the hospital. Before he could intervene, Mrs. Howard reached for her checkbook, and construction of the pool got underway. For two decades members of the board of governors put their stamp on the developing Ochsner Foundation Hospital.

But all the time the board itself was a surplus appendage on the organization chart of the Ochsner Institutions. The governors were originally appointed to lend their efforts solely on behalf of the hospital. The board of trustees had overall control of the Ochsner Foundation and its activities, including the hospital and the education and research programs. When decisions were needed, the trustees made them, whether the hospital or any other foundation operation was involved. At the same time, the affairs of the clinic were administered by the board of management.

No formal line of communication existed between the governors and the trustees or even between the governors and the hospital medical staff, composed of clinic doctors. After a while, the hospital administrator, Horace E. "Sandy" Hamilton, took on the role of the liaison, the go-between. In the early 1970s Hamilton excluded Merrill O. Hines, medical director of the clinic and president of the foundation, and Edgar J. Saux, the clinic's administrative director, from meetings of the board of governors. There wasn't enough space for them in the meeting room, Hamilton explained.

For years the governors gave generously of their time and money to the advancement of the hospital without demanding more than a token voice in the administration of the facility. They found satisfaction enough in watching from close-up seats the explosive development of the Ochsner campus. The laissez-faire attitude changed abruptly, however, with the appointment of five younger New Orleanians to the Board of Governors. The newcomers were Richard W. Freeman, Jr., whose trustee-father was the dominant layman in the foundation after the death of J. Blanc Monroe; Malcolm Monroe's son-in-law J. Thomas Lewis, future president and chairman of the foundation; W. Boatner Reily III; Charles Janvier; and Frederic B. Ingram. They quickly discovered that their position as governors was honorary, and they rebelled.

Hines was summoned one day to the office of the elder Freeman. There he found Freeman, Sr., Freeman, Jr., Reily, and Ingram. The three new governors sounded off. It was ridiculous, they said, for them to waste their time on a board that was nothing more than window dressing. Everybody knew that the clinic doctors ran the Ochsner center. The clinic was a law unto itself, and the foundation was operated by a board of seven trustees, five of whom were second-generation clinic partners. Either there will be changes made, or we will resign from the Board of Governors, the unhappy trio announced. They found sympathetic listeners in Hines and Freeman, Sr., who agreed that the three-board system was outmoded and no longer workable.

The impromptu gathering led to a restructuring of the Alton Ochsner Medical Foundation and a move to redress the balance of administrative power between clinic doctors and volunteer laymen. On June 20, 1973, the Board of Trustees approved the idea of a merger with the Board of Governors. The foundation trustees and the hospital governors met jointly on July 19, 1973, to take the first formal action toward reorganization. They named a committee to work out details of a merger of trustees and governors into a single board with authority to administer the affairs of the foundation.

The young men who had met with Hines—Freeman, Jr., Reily, and Ingram—took seats on the committee along with J. Thomas Lewis, Morrell F. Trimble, William O. Turner, Joseph W. Montgomery, and Richard Freeman, Sr. Merrill Hines and William R. Arrowsmith completed the group. This combination of new blood and experience decided that the trustees and governors should be merged into a single board of trustees to govern all activities of the foundation. Reaching into the past, the committee revived Raymond Rich's recommendation that an executive committee of trustees be created with full authority to act when the entire board was not meeting. In keeping with clinic precedents, the committee decided that no one would be eligible for service on the executive committee after reaching the age of seventy. Attorney Lewis revised the foundation charter to reflect the conditions of the merger, and the trustees adopted the new plan on January 21, 1974.

The executive committee includes fifteen members—eight laymen and seven physicians—thus reversing the makeup of the old board of trustees with its five physicians and two laymen. The executive committee elects both its own members and members of the whole board of trustees. Terms are five years. A member of the executive committee may serve no more than two consecutive terms but is eligible to return to the board after a one-year hiatus, if he is again chosen.

All of the rebellious younger governors were named to the first executive committee of the expanded board of trustees, of which Richard W. Freeman, Sr., became chairman, and the other laymen were Morrell F. Trimble and Malcolm L. Monroe. The seven doctors were William R. Arrowsmith, Paul T. DeCamp, Merrill O. Hines, John C. Weed, C. Thorpe Ray, William D. Davis, Jr., and Thomas E. Weiss.

By 1981 the board of trustees, which had come to serve mostly the advisory functions of a university board of visitors, had sixty-eight members, fifty-one of them nonphysicians. Rich's plan for vesting control in an executive committee was working well.

The reorganization begun in 1972 would seem to have given laymen the edge. They have a narrow numerical advantage over doctors on the executive committee that was set up to manage the foundation and a large majority of seats on the board of trustees. But this should not be seen as a defeat for the clinic doctors. They soon perceived a threat to their position, in the person of the president of the foundation; yet they were easily able to triumph.

In 1973, when Sandy Hamilton, fifth in a line of Ochsner hospital directors after Albert Scheidt, Dr. Lester L. Weissmiller, Dr. Edward Leveroos, and John Rankin, was forced by ill health to ask for retirement, the foundation trustees went hunting for a replacement. They found one and thereby triggered a climactic period in the affairs of foundation and the clinic. The Rush Jordan era will not soon be forgotten in the Jefferson Highway complex. Until Jordan came onto the scene, the clinic partners never felt that their standing in the Ochsner organization was threatened by the lay leadership of the foundation. Now, whether accurately or not, they perceived the new man as an ambitious actor reaching out for a bigger role and shoving the clinic partners to the back of the stage.

To the patient in the Ochsner Foundation Hospital, to the men and women attending Ochsner educational courses, to the researchers in the laboratories, Jordan's fate made no difference. There are successful, efficient medical institutions that are dominated by doctors and others that are controlled by nondoctors. Whatever the result of what turned out to be a one-sided power struggle, the Ochsner center would have remained in business. What was established in the stormy interlude is that for the foreseeable future, Ochsner is a doctors' activity. The founders wouldn't have had it any other way.

The trustees' search committee at first looked for a highly qualified director who could manage a hospital that would soon have a much-expanded capacity. Results were discouraging. Finally, after months of fruitless search, the committee resolved to set its sights higher and seek a professional health field executive who could take on the responsibility of superintending not only the hospital but also the foundation's research and educational programs. In order to attract an outstanding candidate, the trustees decided to offer the presidency of the Alton Ochsner Medical Foundation as part of the job. This approach required Richard Freeman to yield the chairmanship (he became chairman of the finance committee) and Merrill O. Hines to exchange the presidency for the chairman's post. By September, 1974, the executive committee had picked Jack A. Skarupa of Greenville, South Carolina; its long work seemed to be over. But Skarupa suddenly changed his mind and decided to stay in Greenville. He had apparently had his eyes opened to the pitfalls that would lie in the path of any layman who took the job at that time.

One of administrators who had been interviewed earlier was Lemuel Russell "Rush" Jordan, whose background and reputation would command the attention of any head-hunting committee. He had a bachelor's degree from Amherst College and a master's degree from Columbia University. At Duke University and the University of Florida he had served as both medical manager and faculty member. Moving to Birmingham, he was executive director and then president and chief executive officer of the Baptist Medical Center. During Jordan's years there, the Baptist hospitals tripled their capacity, to 930 beds. He was, obviously, one of the talented members of a small cadre of executives who understand the intricacies of the multibillion-dollar business of health care—fund-raising, management, personnel, planning, public relations, and all. The Ochsner searchers were interested, but Jordan asked that his name be withdrawn from consideration. Then, soon after

Skarupa backed out, Jordan telephoned to ask whether the job was still open. The Ochsner trustees heard that he had clashed with the Baptist trustees.

Jordan's troubles at Ochsner began when he came to New Orleans for a final interview, which was more or less a formality, for members of the search committee—especially Richard Freeman—were eager to settle on someone, and Jordan seemed the logical choice. Jordan went to dinner with Freeman and Hines, and they discussed the title that he would have. Hines suggested that Jordan begin as president and chief operating officer, while Hines would serve for the time being as chairman and chief executive officer. Hines said he would yield the chief executive designation to Jordan after the latter had settled into his job. Jordan would have none of this; he insisted on being chief executive officer from the start. Freeman and other members of the search committee overruled Hines and gave Jordan the title he wanted.

Relations between Jordan and Hines were off to a shaky start and deteriorated rapidly. Two hours before Jordan was to appear at a meeting of the trustees for formal election, he went to Hines's office and made a new demand. Jordan said he would have to be named a member of the trustees' executive committee as well as chief executive officer. He noted that the committee exercised the final authority and argued that the president would have to be a member if he were to be effective. "You'll have to talk to Mr. Freeman," Hines responded. After a brief private conference with Freeman, Jordan relented. As president, Jordan was almost constantly at odds with the chairman of the board. He once told Hines, "You've got the worst disposition I've ever seen."

The differences between Jordan and Hines, who was still clinic medical director, might seem just a clash of personalities but actually they were symptomatic of a rift that quickly developed between the new president and some influential doctors in the partnership. There had been only two previous presidents in the three-decade history of the foundation—Alton Ochsner and Merrill Hines—and both were surgeons and stalwarts in the group practice. Neither Blanc Monroe nor Freeman had ever held the title of president. Now here was a rank outsider claiming not only the honors but also the considerable authority that goes with the position. Perhaps a less forceful, less ambitious, more conciliatory executive might have laid out lines of communication with the clinic and eased the tensions. Given Jordan's personality and methods of operation, however, a showdown over control of the Ochsner establishment was certain to occur, and the clinic had the high cards. It was doctors who had founded the New Orleans center, who had provided the patient care, and who had earned the reputation upon which success was built. They would not accept the diminished role for the clinic in future Ochsner activities that Jordan seemed to envision.

Timing worked against Jordan. His stay at Ochsner—from December 1, 1974, until June 29, 1978—coincided with the huge building program that virtually doubled the size of the facilities. When he arrived, Jordan found the fiscal affairs of the foundation in disarray. His first task was to reorganize the activities and assemble a management team. Even his critics credit him with installing a highly efficient system for running the foundation. Yet, while he was devising and implementing the new system, he was also being drawn into making snap decisions about the construction program. By the time the sale of the bond issue allowed work to begin, inflation was causing the cost of construction to soar at an estimated rate of $17,000 a day. The foundation chose to plunge into the work without waiting for blueprints to be completed. Therefore, a building committee that included Jordan had to make decisions and negotiate with the contractor while the walls were rising. Moreover, the building project created an enormously frustrating atmosphere to work in. The pounding of hammers shattered the well-ordered calm of clinic and hospital. Workmen tramped through the halls. Dust drifted into offices, laboratories, patients' rooms. It was human nature to blame someone for the confusion, and Jordan was a highly visible target.

But what eventually proved his undoing was Jordan's apparent inability to understand the unique place held by the clinic in the Ochsner realm. He made some friends in the clinic partnership; yet he ended up with more enemies who distrusted his motives. Almost any layman would have been suspect among the doctors, but a more perceptive newcomer might have sensed the justifiable feeling of proprietorship in the clinic and taken pains to win confidence in his plans.

When Jordan arrived, for example, a sign on the campus identified the Ochsner Medical Center, a name long used to cover all of the activities. In Jordan's time it was replaced with a sign that read, Ochsner Medical Institutions. The new designation was perhaps more descriptive of the functions and was approved by Alton Ochsner himself; nevertheless, it raised questions among the doctors. As some of them saw it, Jordan was treating each of the activities on the campus as that of a separate institution. If this were true, the clinic, instead of being the coequal of the foundation, would be downgraded to rank with Brent House, the Richard W. Freeman Research Institute, the school for technologists, and other elements.

The fears were reinforced when Jordan took the lead in bringing about a merger on May 3, 1976, of the foundation and the Eye, Ear, Nose, and Throat Hospital, later the Louisiana Eye and Ear Institute, in New Orleans. Ochsner had been approached by the board of trustees of the eye hospital, which was having financial difficulties. Under Jordan's leadership, the hospital began to flourish, with the help of economies such as joint bulk purchasing with the Ochsner Foundation Hospital. Jordan also promoted valuable support for the Eye Institute from the Lions Club and the New Orleans Saints professional football club. However, the merger was received with no great enthusiasm by some in the clinic. The agreement provided for an open staff at the Eye and Ear Institute, that is, any doctor who could qualify professionally would be eligible to practice there. The foundation was moving into new territory without taking the clinic along.

Jordan talked about the provision of management services to hospitals far afield. He sent an aide to San José, Costa Rica, in 1976 for preliminary discussions with a group of physicians who proposed to open an Ochsner-like clinic and hospital. And there were feelers from the financially ailing Atlanta West General Hospital in Georgia.

At home, he led a group of Ochsner physicians in an inspection of the Sara Mayo Hospital, now the New Orleans General Hospital, after its board suggested that a merger be studied. Discussions did not get very far, but in 1978 a call for help from the board of the Crippled Children's Hospital, now the Children's Hospital, pulled the foundation into a public controversy. Strapped for funds, the Children's Hospital board reached a preliminary agreement with an Ochsner committee that included Richard Freeman, Jordan, and clinic medical director Frank A. Riddick, Jr. The plan was for Ochsner to move its pediatric practice to Children's, which would continue to have an open staff arrangement. But some of the Children's doctors rebelled. They described Ochsner as an octopus, stretching its tentacles to snare as many area hospitals as it could. Octopus was the word some clinic partners used for Jordan himself. The dissident Children's staff doctors finally managed to block any affiliation.

What was not clear to skeptical partners is what position the clinic would occupy if the foundation became involved in the operation of hospitals in addition Ochsner itself. Where would the expansion path lead in the end?

Other developments over which Jordan had no control made it appear to his critics that he was discriminating against the clinic. When the foundation took over the radiology department in order to finance new equipment, some of the partners considered the deal to be a steal from the clinic. Other partners were angered when the foundation increased the rent charged for the clinic building nearly fivefold when the five-story addition was completed as part of the overall expansion project. Jordan had nothing to do with the increase but took much of the blame nevertheless. Freeman recalls that he himself felt some coolness as a result of the new rent scale. A clue to the tensions can be seen in the fact that the clinic ceased making annual contributions to the foundation after the rent increased.

Six months after he took office, Jordan might have anticipated better relations with the clinic when the age restriction required Hines to step aside as medical director and Frank Riddick was elected. At first Riddick was supportive.

When he had been at Ochsner for about a year, Jordan went to see Riddick one day. He said that at his age he felt there was still time for him to make one more change in jobs if it appeared advantageous from the standpoint of his career. He asked Riddick to make a frank evaluation of his performance as president. Taken by surprise, Riddick replied that he would need time to think it over, that he would respond later.

Months passed. Riddick continued to defend Jordan, to act as a buffer between the president and doctors who were disenchanted. But the medical director and member of the trustees' executive committee gradually concluded that Jordan's actions were divisive, that he was causing a polarization of loyalties between foundation and clinic.

The event that moved Riddick to a decision was Jordan's effort to establish a planning division with a director who would function as a member of Jordan's executive staff. The rub was that Jordan wanted the clinic to bear half the division's expenses. Riddick and other members of the board of management felt the clinic would not have enough voice in an activity Jordan would dominate to justify the cost to the partnership. Actually, Riddick had come to the realization that the board would reject any joint project involving foundation and clinic. Before the clinic's veto stalled Jordan's project, David R. Pitts was interviewed as a prospective planning director. Jordan eventually hired him as hospital administrator.

His mind made up, Riddick sought an appointment with Jordan. "You asked me several months ago whether I thought you had a future at Ochsner," Riddick said to Jordan. "I am ready now to tell you. I think you have an important contribution to make to American health care, but I believe you should make it somewhere else." Riddick said, in effect, that Jordan's usefulness at Ochsner had ended. Later, Riddick said he had expected Jordan to land another job and to make a graceful exit from New Orleans by announcing at the impending dedication of the expanded campus facilities that he had fulfilled his assignment here and was moving on to a new challenge. But Jordan was not prepared to depart without a fight. "The medical director just fired me," he said by way of opening a telephone conversation with trustee J. Thomas Lewis.

Once the break with Riddick was out in the open, Jordan's tenure was headed for an abrupt end. Freeman and Lewis asked Jordan to meet them in Lewis's office at the law firm of Monroe and Lemann, scene of so many sessions in the clinic's early years. They told Jordan the trustees would be generous, but he would have to leave. Jordan said it would be easier to find another employer while he still had a job, and it was agreed that he could remain as president for several months while he made a search.

Unwilling to fade quietly from the scene, Jordan turned against Pitts, whom the executive committee had promoted to executive vice-president of the foundation. Jordan believed Pitts had eyes on the presidency. He presented the executive committee with charges of misconduct against the vice-president. At a meeting held in an office of the clinic building in order to preserve secrecy, the committee delved into the accusations, and absolved Pitts on every count. Under the circumstances, either Jordan or Pitts had to go, and it was Jordan. Lewis walked over to Jordan's office in the Libby-Dufour Building. He told Jordan that his salary would continue until the end of the year and he could keep the automobile provided by the foundation but that he was to clear out his desk and leave Ochsner that day. Jordan was elected president of the Eye and Ear Institute, which was soon to regain its independence from Ochsner, and managed the facility until he moved to a job in Dayton, Ohio.

CHAPTER THIRTEEN

The Third Generation

In 1978 the executive committee of the trustees turned to a layman, one of its own number, to salve the wounds left over from the Rush Jordan era. On June 29 they chose attorney J. Thomas Lewis as interim president and chief executive officer of the Alton Ochsner Medical Foundation. Son-in-law of the longtime trustee Malcolm L. Monroe and a partner in the law firm of Monroe and Lemann, Lewis had experience in Ochsner affairs as a legal advisor and a member of the former board of governors as well as the board of trustees. With his well-developed powers of persuasion and his low-key, conciliatory approach, Lewis proved to be the kind of executive that was needed to relax the strains that had developed between foundation and clinic personnel and to ease the adjustment to the greatly expanded facilities.

One of the younger members of the group of New Orleans business and professional leaders who have devoted much of their public activity to the Ochsner cause, Lewis became involved with the institutions soon after he began to practice law. The son of a naval officer, he was born at Long Beach, California, October 15, 1936. He was graduated cum laude from Princeton University in 1959, served a hitch with the United States Navy Reserves, then entered the Tulane law school. He has been president of the board of trustees of the New Orleans Museum of Art and has held membership on the board of the Eye and Ear Institute of Louisiana. As one of the nonpolitical members of the Board of Liquidation, City Debt, he has represented the public in keeping an eye on the borrowing practices of the city of New Orleans.

Lewis remembers his presidency of the Ochsner Foundation as "a

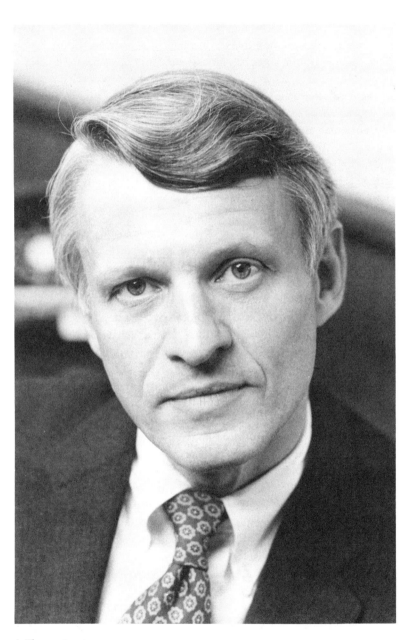
J. Thomas Lewis

piece of cake." "For one thing, everybody knew I was temporary. I was not seen as a threat," he explains. He made it plain in accepting the job that it would not be a permanent assignment because he did not want to abandon his career in law. Besides, he felt that "a doctor has status in the medical world, and a layman cannot have the same standing." Nevertheless, his performance pleased his fellow trustees, including the physician members, and he could have continued had he been willing.

The logical time for installing a new president was May 1, 1980, when age regulations would require Merrill O. Hines to retire as chairman of the trustees, opening up a spot in which Lewis could continue his close connections with the foundation without having to spend full time at these duties. In August, 1979, Lewis told members of the medical staff and division heads of the foundation that the time had come to begin a search for a permanent president. He polled them on their ideas about the qualifications that the new chief executive officer should possess. As for educational background, 46 respondents said he should be a medical doctor, 26 said he should have the degree of master of business administration, 8 replied that he should have an M.D. plus a supplemental degree, and 29 expressed no preference. In the matter of experience and training, 46 opted for business administration, 90 for health-care administration, 18 for the practice of medicine, and 10 for medical education. Asked about a background of employment within the Ochsner Institutions, 13 thought it extremely important, 20 very important, 33 slightly important and 43 not important.

Richard Freeman became chairman of a search committee that included four lay and four physician members. One of the committee's decisions was that the foundation should first try to find a doctor who could carry out the president's duties and that the hunt should first be made within the Ochsner walls. The joint policy committee of the clinic and foundation, of which Frank Riddick was chairman, concurred in this approach and also recommended that a physician-president continue to practice medicine part-time. There were echoes from the Jordan regime in the agreement that the president of the foundation should sit in on the meetings of the clinic's board of management, although he would have no vote. Freeman had emphasized in the discussions that the foundation "is not a separate entity but is a partner in a team effort embracing Ochsner Clinic as a full partner."

Riddick let it be known at first that he would be interested in the presidency. Without question, he would have had the backing of the clinic partnership. But Freeman reminded Riddick that as medical director he already held the most powerful post on the campus, and his departure might upset the smooth functioning of the clinic. Riddick finally concluded that although the foundation offered an intriguing challenge, a sideways move was not sufficiently inviting. Once Riddick pulled out, he joined with Freeman as a two-man subcommittee for selecting a nominee to present to the executive committee of the trustees.

One of the supporters of the Riddick candidacy was George H. Porter III. Once Riddick was out of the race, Porter listened when Lewis sounded him out for the post. He asked for a week to think it over, and then he said he would serve if the presidency were offered. He was elected by the executive committee and assumed office on May 1, 1980, the fifth president of the foundation in succession to medical doctors Alton Ochsner and Merrill Hines and laymen Jordan and Lewis. Lewis moved up to chairman.

For the first time in thirty-eight years of Ochsner activity, the full leadership became the responsibility of internists. Riddick, of course, had been medical director of the clinic for five years, but throughout that period Merrill Hines, a colon and rectal surgeon, was an active and influential chairman of the foundation. Before then, surgeons predominated in both clinic and foundation.

Riddick and Porter brought similar backgrounds to their Ochsner affiliations. Both are southerners, Riddick having been born at Memphis on June 14, 1929, and Porter at Charlotte, North Carolina, on September 7, 1933. Both are honor graduates of highly regarded southern universities and medical schools. Riddick obtained his cum laude bachelor of arts degree from Vanderbilt University in 1951 and his medical degree from the Vanderbilt School of Medicine in 1954. Porter earned his magna cum laude bachelor of arts degree at Duke University in 1954 and his doctor of medicine diploma from Duke in 1958. Both were tapped for coveted membership in the Alpha Omega Alpha honorary medical fraternity. Both had experience in medical re-

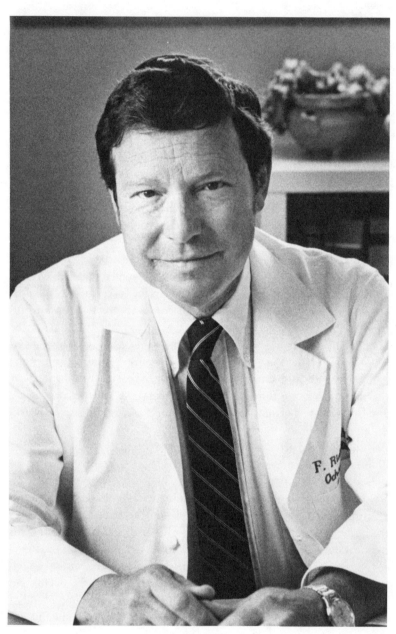

Frank A. Riddick, Jr.

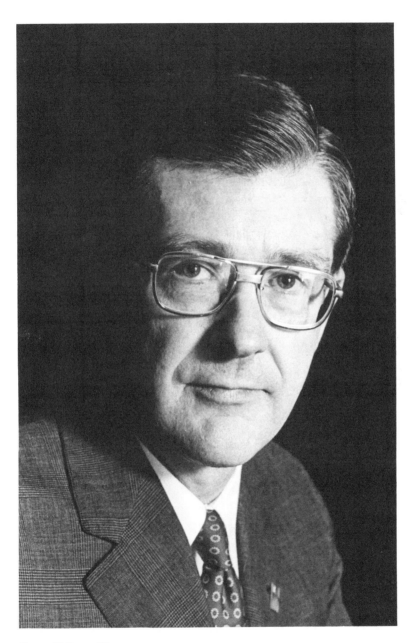

George H. Porter III

search early in their careers, and both showed an interest in administration after joining the Ochsner staff.

Their paths first converged in 1959 when Porter became an assistant resident in medicine at the Barnes Hospital, St. Louis. After his internship at Barnes, Riddick had spent two years as an army doctor before returning to Barnes. He took over as chief resident in medicine during the year Porter was an assistant. Both have painful memories of one event in their year together. They were making the hospital rounds with a visiting internist when one of the accompanying Barnes doctors collapsed from a heart attack. Riddick and Porter worked over him for two hours in a vain attempt to revive him.

Riddick, an endocrinologist, remained in St. Louis for the 1960–1961 academic year as a fellow in medicine, studying metabolic disease at the Washington University School of Medicine. He had ideas of a life in the laboratory until gradually he reached the conclusion that "I was a pretty lousy rat doctor and a pretty good human doctor." He sought an interview with William R. Arrowsmith, the chief of medicine at Ochsner, and went to work on July 1, 1961.

Porter, a hematologist, completed his internship at the Duke Medical Center before joining Riddick at Barnes. He next became senior resident physician at the Peter Bent Brigham Hospital at Boston, an affiliate of the Harvard Medical School. His interest in research led him to a three-year assignment as a fellow in hematology at the National Institutes of Health, Bethesda, Maryland. Just as Riddick had done, Porter decided that he wanted to be a teacher and to treat patients. He talked with Riddick about Ochsner. "The fact that Frank was happy here told me that it was a grand institution." Arrowsmith and Hines hired Porter in April, 1964.

Neither Riddick nor Porter decided to go into medicine until he was already in college. Riddick as a teenager wanted to be a lawyer. He was skilled in debate as a student and has never lost the advocate's way with words. His knack for dissecting the elements of a problem and clarifying the alternatives has been one of his strengths in management councils. He chose to take biology in college only because a course was offered at a convenient time. Once he had a sample of science, he was hooked. Porter, as an undergraduate at Duke, was torn between business and medicine. In early semesters he took some courses that would prepare him for medical school and others that would qualify him to enter the business administration school. He finally opted for medicine. Merrill Hines received a head injury in an automobile collision on the River Road on Labor Day, 1967, and Alton Ochsner awakened to the fact that the clinic had not trained anyone to take over in the event the medical director should die or be disabled. "We have got to do something," Ochsner exclaimed. Even if there were no unexpected vacancy, the time had come to establish a succession, for Hines would have to retire in 1975. Founder Edgar Burns was named chairman of a committee charged with selecting one or two assistant medical directors who could be groomed to become the clinic's chief executive officer. The Burns committee settled upon Riddick and gynecologist William L. Geary, and the board of management appointed them. Geary did not take to the administrative routine and soon stepped aside. Riddick, on the other hand, enjoyed being in on decision making. "Power is pretty heady," he confesses. And he found Hines to be a good teacher. By 1972, when he was promoted to associate medical director and already recognized as the crown prince, Riddick had realized that the directorship would allow him to practice medicine only part-time. Later, when he was medical director, he would philosophize: "There's a real challenge in running this place. If I can somehow guide and lead this group into doing great things in delivering medical care, then I may have magnified my ability to treat patients."

Riddick and Porter were both active in the maneuvering among younger physicians that resulted in adoption of the revised clinic partnership agreement of 1971. They were members of the committee chosen to draft what is essentially the constitution that governs the clinic, and Riddick was the principal author. In 1975 he was nominated by the board of management and elected medical director. He became a trustee of the foundation in 1973 and a member of the executive committee of the trustees in 1977.

The events of a January day in 1978 demonstrate some of the reasons why the clinic has prospered under Riddick's direction. He and his wife, the former Mary Belle Alston, were in a downtown bank office arranging for a mortgage to finance their new home when an overwhelming feeling of weakness alerted the physician that he was having a severe heart attack. Assisted to a sofa in an vice-president's office, he directed his wife to call an ambulance and conferred on her a power of attorney in order that the mortgage transaction could be completed despite his illness. In the ambulance he reached up from a stretcher and turned on a flow of oxygen that the attendant had not started. When the attendant told the driver that she could find no blood pressure or pulse, Riddick remarked that there had to be pressure because he was talking. He counted his own pulse—a rate of forty—and noted the sharp chest pains that confirmed a myocardial infarction. He instructed the driver to pass up nearer hospitals and take him directly to Ochsner. Cardiologists there waited for the arrival of the ambulance, but heart surgeon Noel L. Mills, summoned from his home, was halted on the River Road by a stalled freight train. He abandoned his automobile on the side of the road, climbed between boxcars, and raced on foot the rest of the way to the hospital. Charles B. Moore and Fortune A. Dugan stayed at the bedside for forty-eight hours until Riddick was out of danger. Even during illness, Riddick was in command.

Guy Caldwell and Merrill Hines had reached out and collected enough responsibility to make the medical director the most powerful member of the clinic staff, but each had ruled on an ad hoc basis. When Riddick began writing the terms of the 1971 partnership, he knew that if events took their expected course, he would succeed to the office in 1975. He was, in effect, drawing up the specifications for his own future job. His experience as an assistant convinced him that the director had to have authority, and he embedded in the agreement provision for prerogatives that had been enjoyed before partly by custom and partly by the persuasiveness of his predecessors. Caldwell and Hines served by election of the board of management. Riddick changed that plan and provided for election of the director by the entire partnership. Once elected, he serves an indefinite term. Riddick considered the alternative of requiring the incumbent to stand for reelection at intervals. As it is, the director is spared periodic politicking and can make decisions without worrying about his popularity. He is by no means an absolute monarch, however, since he can be dethroned at any time by the vote of four members of the seven-man board of administrators. The sources of the director's power lie in the fact that he draws up the agendas for meetings of the board, that he serves on the major administrative committees, that management communications are routed through his office, and that he practices medicine only two half-days a week and has more time than the other partners to stay well informed about problems affecting the institutions. The board of management has the ultimate authority. It is much more an executive than a legislative body. And the medical director serves as the board's ex officio chairman.

Riddick has no cat-o'-nine-tails in his office—wouldn't know how to wield it if he did. The 109 partners and 75 staff doctors cannot be flogged into line. They have to be led by persuasion, convinced that a course of action is logical. It is an approach made to order for Riddick's style. He takes the time to examine the ramifications of a problem, outlines the alternatives, and advances the arguments for the solutions that he suggests. Most of his persuasion is done in informal discussions. Because he feels that he cannot take strong advocacy positions while presiding at meetings of the board of management, Riddick makes his views known in advance.

Riddick notes that the challenge of his job is to create an effective medical organization, "and it's not too different from being a practitioner. It's political in a way. Sometimes in dealing with a patient it's clear what needs to be done, but the patient has to be persuaded." In the same way, the staff must often be sold on a course of action the advantages of which are apparent to the director. Riddick delegates business management to the administrative director, Francis Manning, but leads in the decision making when the practice of medicine is involved. "I try not to run a complaint department, but if I try to delegate this function, it comes back to me in the end anyway." Personnel problems usually stem from individual inertia or from the occasional maverick who upsets the teamwork functioning on which group practice is based. Riddick prefers to handle these situations through department or section heads.

The more than doubling of the size of the staff in recent years came at a cost of some of the camaraderie that existed in the 1960s. Riddick's door is open to any doctor who wants to see him. He eats lunch every day in the staff section of the cafeteria, circulates at social functions, and attends every board or committee meeting when he is in New Orleans. At Ochsner there is none of the stuffiness that sometimes marks the relationships among senior and junior members of medical school faculties. The numbers prevent the director from scheduling periodic interviews with partners and staff members, but the organization nevertheless is not so big that Riddick cannot know who is having a family crisis, who is unhappy and preparing to leave, who is making strides professionally.

The usually affable Riddick does get angry over what he considers unjust criticism of the clinic administration by a partner, based on the latter's own perception of a problem. Often Riddick responds by dictating a sarcastic memorandum. Usually he puts the document aside overnight and then tears it up. "It's a sort of catharsis. It's one of the things I learned from Dr. Arrowsmith." But Riddick will bring on a showdown if he is pushed to it.

Sports-minded practitioners and employees learned that they sometimes could make a profit by betting on "Dr. Riddick." That is the name given to a racehorse by one of the director's patients, Albert Stall. The thoroughbred was a successful campaigner at the Fairgrounds in New Orleans and other tracks as well.

By the time George Porter was admitted into the clinic partnership in 1967, he realized that he had found at Ochsner a rare opportunity for a career in which he could combine his twin interests of medicine and business administration. He became one of the younger staff members who rebelled against the dominance of the old-timers entrenched on the self-perpetuating board of management. He joined Riddick on the committee that rewrote the partnership agreement of 1957, and the revision of 1971 also reflects his thinking. His prominence in the uprising led to his membership on the board of management beginning in 1973 as the second partner to be elected under the new democratic formula after urologist William Brannan. By the time Porter's seven-year term expired on April 30, 1980—the day before he took office as president of the foundation—he understood the workings of the clinic as few members ever did. "He used to drive the [business] staff crazy with his questions," recalled Ed Saux, who predicted at the time a bright presidency for Porter. "He's smart."

The job has turned out to be rewarding and satisfying even beyond Porter's expectations. Stepping in without previous administrative experience to become chief executive officer of a $2-million-a-week business was a test of his acumen, but Porter learned as he went along. A do-it-yourself perfectionist, he soon discovered that he had to delegate authority, but he dislikes unpleasant surprises and insists on being kept informed. "I like to know the details. You can look at the big picture, but you'd better understand the details, too." Beneath a suave exterior is a cool resolve. "If you can't bear to fire somebody, you don't belong in an executive's job." An early casualty of the Porter administration was the foundation's executive vice-president and hospital director, David R. Pitts.

Porter prizes cordial community relations as one of Ochsner's strengths and is conscious of his position as the most visible representative of the institutions off the campus. A member of the exclusive clubs, as Ochsner leaders have been since the time of the founders, he also is a director of the Hibernia National Bank, the Chamber of Commerce, and the Metropolitan Crime Commission. He enjoys social occasions. As president, he understands the pervasive role that government—national, state, and local—plays in health activities and has not neglected his contacts with public officials. "You've got to have political savvy. You've got to be able to see the governor when it's necessary."

The previous practitioner-presidents, Alton Ochsner and Merrill Hines, were long-hour, nose-to-the-grindstone workers, and Porter is no clock-watcher, either. After an eleven-hour day on the campus, he takes reports and studies home for a couple of hours of after-dinner thinking—synthesizing and analyzing, as he calls it. It's a time when he can be alone. He and his wife, Virginia Pillow Porter, an anesthesiologist and partner in the clinic, have tacitly agreed not to burden each other with their individual professional problems. They met in 1951 when as undergraduates they worked side by side in a Duke University laboratory. They began dating as sophomores in the Duke medical school and were married in their senior year.

A violinist who used to play with amateur string groups, Porter occasionally finds time to tune up for his own amusement. He likes to listen to music and tapes selections that interest him. He enjoys Mozart, and thinks this is an indication of his basic conservatism. "I feel comfortable with the classic mode." He repairs and maintains antique clocks, and he and his wife are collectors of furniture. "A damn good chef," he nevertheless manages to keep his weight at 160 pounds. He gardens and does yard work. "I'd never be bored."

When Porter moved over to the foundation, his membership in the clinic was put into a trust over which he has no control. He continues to see patients part-time at the clinic, but the compensation goes directly to the foundation. He draws no pay from the institutions except his foundation salary.

George Porter wants to be remembered as the president who kept the foundation strong in the fields of education and research. "We have to manage our resources carefully. I want to be a steward of the purse, but I am not the superconservative watchdog some people think I am. I simply believe in conserving assets so as to fulfill goals. We have to watch our money." Yet, he makes it plain, the foundation will not balance its budget at the expense of education and research.

CHAPTER FOURTEEN

Research at Ochsner's

Ochsner employees call the complex on the Jefferson Highway a campus, and they are not putting on airs. The cluster of buildings is a seat of learning and scientific research, as well as a center of healing. Educational activities equal those of a small university in scope and diversity.

Beginning in 1944, the founders were willing to dip into their limited assets in order to fulfill what they saw as an obligation to their profession. They eagerly borrowed the ideas of medicine's innovators in order to treat their own patients more efficiently. They enlisted low-paid trainees to help them run the hospital that they were planning. Now, once they could see their way clear financially, it was time for them to begin aiding the search for scientific discoveries that they could share with other practitioners and using their teaching skills to prepare young doctors who would go out to take care of the sick. Professors themselves, the five realized that the eventual success of their enterprise depended on research and education, as well as patient care. Nineteen years later, an ad hoc committee of doctors who were invited to look over Ochsner's research functions and make suggestions summed up the founders' thinking. "The patients of the Ochsner Clinic receive superior medical care," wrote the committee in its report. "Good medical practice might continue for many years without associated research, but the committee believes the practice would be more local in geography and more general in nature. The place which the Ochsner Clinic and Foundation will occupy nationally and internationally in medicine in the years to come and the distances from which patients and scholars will be attracted to it, will be determined by the quality of research and educational programs which the Clinic and Foundation superimpose upon the superior practice of medicine."

The commitment never wavered. Through lean years and good, the management always found a way to keep training interns and residents and supporting scientists in the Ochsner laboratories. In 1982 the clinic board of management and foundation trustees reaffirmed their intent in a statement of mission that concluded:

> In *Medical Education*, the Institutions will emphasize the importance of academic training in the provision of high quality care through:
> - programs of post graduate physician and allied health professional education
> - continuing education programs for professional staff, Institution employees, and the regional medical community
> - participation, in conjunction with medical schools, in undergraduate medical education
> - patient and public education
>
> In *Research*, a number of basic and clinically oriented research projects will be undertaken to enhance medical knowledge and the Institutions' commitment to a total program of medical care development. The scope of research is consonant with the resources of the Institutions and complements the clinical interests of the physicians of the group.

In the restless tides of humanity that surge through the corridors of the Ochsner buildings are hundreds of men and women who come to learn. They range in age from the late teens to the sixties because the educational program is wide-ranging and attracts enrollees of different levels of attainment. The oldest group includes practicing physicians who converge from all over the United States to attend continuing education programs. The more than twelve hundred practitioners who enroll annually receive credit from the American Medical Association and the American Academy of Family Practice for taking update courses offered by the Ochsner staff.

Ever since the creation of the foundation in 1944 Ochsner has offered fellowships—internships and residencies—to new medical school graduates who get their graduate training and begin their preparation for their specialty practices. Even before the foundation was organized, the clinic took on a small squad of rotating residents for training under a program in which the Tulane medical school and Charity Hospital cooperated. The first to make his appearance, on November 1, 1942, was Harry G. Brown of Florence, Alabama. He was invited to have lunch with the staff in the library and, by chance, sat next to Willoughby E. Kittredge. After they had eaten, Kittredge invited Brown to look over the urology department. "I handed him a white coat and put him to work, and that is how the first Ochsner fellow became a urologist," Kittredge recalled. Brown went back to his hometown to practice his specialty. Since the first class entered the program then directed by Dean H. Echols, Ochsner has sent out nearly fourteen hundred fellows who have equipped themselves to take their board examinations and qualify as specialists. They have spread out over many parts of the country and some foreign areas, and some have been tapped for membership on the Ochsner staff. Since most settle in the institutions' drawing territory, it is true that Ochsner has trained some of its own competition.

In any year there are about two hundred fellows. They are the white-coated doctors who help take care of patients in the hospital and who assist senior staff members in the clinic. Residents are enrolled in twenty-eight specialty training programs, which may be as short as two years or as long as six. As the seniors complete their training and move on, their places are taken by new classes. Recruitment is done through a nationwide computer program in which the choices of training institutions are matched against the selections by medical school graduates. About half of Ochsner's fellows earned membership in Alpha Omega Alpha, the honorary medical fraternity, which takes in only honor students. The Ochsner residents rotate through a period of seeing patients in the South Louisiana Medical Center at Houma.

Another phase of the educational program is the instruction of junior and senior medical school students, most of them from Tulane and Louisiana State University, who spend part of their time at the hospital. The foundation also trains many of its technicians through its School of Allied Health Sciences. Courses are offered in blood bank technology, dietetics, health care administration, medical technology, nuclear medicine technology, radiologic therapy, respiratory technology, surgical technology, ultrasound technology, and extracorporeal technology (heart-lung machine operation.) A clinic staff doctor is coordinator for each of the technical courses, and David R. Page, hospital director, and Francis F. Manning, clinic administrative director, are preceptors of the health administration program. Jill Spillane and Sara Crumley direct the dietetic courses.

"Ochsner University" has no football team, no bands, no cheerleaders, but it provides educational opportunity for several hundred undergraduate, graduate, and postgraduate students. The program is supported by the foundation, which depends partly upon contributions from donors.

The foundation's research program dates back to July 11, 1944, when the trustees approved the hiring of Dr. and Mrs. Otto Schales as directors of the investigative laboratory. The chemists were recruited, at $300 a month for Dr. Schales and $200 for his wife, from the Peter Bent Brigham Hospital at Boston. They set up Ochsner's first research laboratory on the second floor of the former Denegre Martin residence on Prytania Street next door to the main clinic building and began doing basic research in chemistry. One of their major interests was in the properties of renin, an enzyme found in the kidney.

Ochsner's longtime involvement in research on the diagnosis and treatment of breast cancer began in 1945 with the employment of Albert Segaloff as head of endocrine research. Segaloff set up a laboratory of his own in the Martin building and enclosed a second-story porch, in which he installed the valuable colonies of rats that he had acquired while he was still a student at Wayne State University. The rats were vital assets in his study of the effects of hormones on breast cancers. They were later moved to cages on the roof of the main clinic building. In 1959 the research activities were transferred to the new campus and installed in the building of what is now the Richard Freeman Research Institute. While the cages were being lowered from the roof of the old clinic building, a cable broke. Scores of the animals were killed in the five-story fall. The accident wiped out a study of colon cancer in which Segaloff also was engaged. But he still had his breeding stock, and his unique colonies survive.

A practitioner in the clinic as well as a researcher, Segaloff has been a pioneer in the application of research findings to the treatment of patients. He arranged for one of the first adrenalectomies (surgical removal of the adrenal glands) in 1953, producing dramatic shrinkage in the breast tumor of a Biloxi, Mississippi, patient, although she died

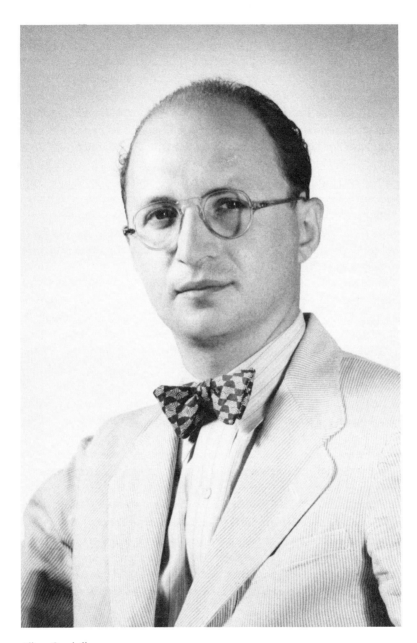

Albert Segaloff

because the disease had already spread. Patients can survive without the adrenals when they are treated with cortisone. In 1951 he published the first paper on the treatment of breast cancer with testosterone. He has sounded repeated warnings about routine mammography, X-ray examination of the breast, which carries a high risk of inducing cancer. Segaloff has been recognized internationally for his development of a standard for measuring breast tumors. His method lets investigators know precisely what effect a method of treatment has on a tumor—whether it works or not. In 1955 Segaloff published a landmark paper on the treatment of adrenal hyperplasia—virilism—with cortisone. The therapy enables some victims to bear children and prevents the growth of moustaches and development of masculine voices. In 1976 he received a $476,404 research contract from the National Cancer Institute to study the influence of repeated low-dose radiation on breast cancer in rats.

In 1976 Edward D. Frohlich brought his team from the University of Oklahoma, and the foundation began a major research effort in hypertension—high blood pressure. Frohlich came in as vice-president in charge of education and research. While he was a staff member of the research division of the Cleveland Clinic from 1964 until 1969, Frohlich became the first practitioner in the United States to use propalonol in the treatment of hypertension. The drug already had been approved in England and, since Frohlich's pioneering, has become the leading beta-blocking agent prescribed in this country. His interest in hypertension quickened, he moved to Oklahoma in 1969 and organized a group of investigators. He had a bid to take his associates to the Mayo Clinic but elected to transfer to Ochsner instead. The foundation's emergence as one of the major centers of research was marked in 1980 by the choice of New Orleans as the site of the first meeting in the United States of the International Society of Hypertension. Of 128 research presentations made to the twelve hundred delegates from forty countries, Ochsner scientists presented 8. Of 35 papers on high blood pressure read at the 1982 meeting of the American Heart Association, 3 were from Ochsner. The foundation's work clearly was winning recognition.

As set up by Frohlich, Ochsner's program involves an examination of the clinical experience to determine which treatments had been the most effective. Charts are reviewed for what they may reveal, and in the laboratory, researchers study blood cells and examine such variables as blood pressures and urine flow. They also make models of the disease to learn the response to various drugs. And finally, the Ochsner group has been chosen by pharmaceutical companies to test new drugs. "We're on the cutting edge," Frohlich explains. "We are able to give our patients the benefit of improved drugs long before they come onto the market generally. We were early with Atenolol, Captopril, and Enalopril, for instance."

Staff members of the clinic are engaged in their own research projects, which are supported by Frohlich's department. Ochsner physicians developed a means of measuring the chemical substance oxalate in the blood, laying groundwork that may eventually allow physicians to inhibit the formation of kidney stones. Surgeons are looking into new treatments for peptic and stress ulcers and for shock. Ophthalmologists have developed new medical therapy for glaucoma. Psychiatrists are learning more about brain chemicals that may cause depression. Rudolph H. Ehrensing, head of psychiatry, collaborated in a study of peptide hormones and their potential in the diagnosis and treatment of emotional disorders. His partner was Andrew V. Schally of New Orleans, co-winner in 1977 of the Nobel Prize in medicine for another project.

CHAPTER FIFTEEN

A Great Hospital Faces the Future

"Worn out joints can now be replaced, narrowed or clogged arteries can be bypassed, electric pacemakers can restore health v.hen the heartbeat has become irregular or erratic, high blood pressure is effectively treated, transplanted kidneys or machines restore function, and many cancers are either curable or controlled." So did President George H. Porter III sum up the major therapeutic advances that had occurred since the founders had launched their clinic forty years earlier. The scientific and surgical achievements of the four decades rivaled in their benefits the development of the sulfa drugs and penicillin and other antibiotics, which already had begun to brighten the outlook for mankind by the time the clinic opened. Revolutionary though they are, the new treatments are no more far-reaching than the changes that also have taken place in the economics of health care, the delivery of medical services, and the operation of hospitals. The environment in which the third generation of leadership of the Ochsner Institutions must compete bears little similarity to the scene Alton Ochsner and his partners entered in 1942. The founders had the advantage of a wartime shortage of physicians, as well as a dearth throughout the Deep South of specialists to whom practitioners could refer their problem patients. At the time they opened their first hospital, there was an acute lack of beds in New Orleans. The developmental phase of the institutions coincided with the period when the federal government, employers, and insurance companies were financing ever more generous patient entitlements.

By the time Porter, Frank A. Riddick, Jr., and new trustees and members of the board of management inherited the responsibility for guiding the institutions, they had to find their way around in a different medical world. The number of active physicians in the United States had almost tripled according to American Medical Association statistics showing 165,290 in 1940 against 450,112 in 1981. In 1940 only one in five doctors—36,880 altogether—was a specialist; by 1981 the ratio had been reversed, and there were 370,151 specialists, four out of five of the doctors who were practicing. In forty-one years the number of generalists, including those in family practice, actually had declined by more than half, from 128,410 to 60,594. These are the doctors who refer patients to specialists. The surge to specialization had barely begun in 1950 when Guy A. Caldwell was already blaming a temporary falling off in the clinic's work load on "the considerable increase in the number of doctors and competent specialists who have established themselves in the small centers throughout our drawing territory." The implications for a clinic that had been established as court of last resort for referred patients, a center for tertiary care, are no less unmistakable now than they were when Caldwell was writing. The Executive Planning Council, made up of key managers from both clinic and foundation, has to look ahead with the knowledge that the Graduate Education National Advisory Committee projects a 43 percent increase in the number of physicians in the United States by 1990. An oversupply of practitioners, most of them specialists, can only mean more competition.

Eleven private hospitals in New Orleans had a total of barely 2,000 beds in 1947. But the drive to provide more facilities, beginning in the 1950s, left the area overbedded. In 1982 there were 6,088 beds in twenty-five hospitals, in addition to the 1,125 that Charity Hospital of Louisiana still maintained for the needy. Even though the available facilities were not being utilized to capacity, another 680 beds were being planned for completion by 1985. The competition from conventional hospitals was going to be intensified, but the planners also had to deal with the emergence of such patient-snaring enterprises as emergency care centers, ambulatory surgical centers, commercial laboratories, mobile diagnostic centers, birthing centers, and home health care services. Louisiana became one of seven states where profit-making, investor-owned chains concentrated their efforts, and by 1982 there were forty-two proprietary hospitals with more than 4,100 beds in Ochsner's home state. By confining their activities to the more lucrative patient services and avoiding costly educational and research projects, the proprietary centers earn dividends for their investors. They compete with nonprofit hospitals, such as Ochsner, which must provide the full gamut of care and at the same time train future practitioners and contribute to the development of medical science.

In the early 1980s the rain of gold on American health care activities began to turn into a drizzle. President Ronald Reagan, who took office in 1981, started his promised reduction of federal expenditures on social programs, among them Medicare and Medicaid. It was the year in which the total cost of health services for the first time exceeded 10 percent of the gross national product. Coincidentally, in the same year the General Motors Corporation spent an average of $3,270 for each employee on health insurance premiums. Industry, paying as fringe benefits about one-third of the total bill for employee health programs, began exploring means of retrenching. Insurance companies were caught in a squeeze between ever-increasing costs and the resistance of customers to higher premiums. One solution was to make the patient bear a greater portion of doctor and hospital fees by raising the deductibles. Both government and employers also began balking at paying for unnecessary services. Panels made up of knowledgeable professionals began to scrutinize statements, and reimbursement was refused for questionable items. Was a patient kept in the hospital for five days when he could have safely been sent home after three days? Could a surgical procedure have been done on an ambulatory basis? The burden was placed on practitioners to defend their decisions. Medicare and Medicaid payments were based on established norms. Because of restrictions placed by the government, Medicare patients no longer contributed their share of the costs of peripheral activities, such as doctor training. The load was shifted to private patients at a time when the aged population is in the process of doubling, as it is expected to do in fifty years, and Medicare patients will claim an increasing share of hospital beds.

With hospital expenses zooming at a rate of almost 20 pecent a year, various plans aimed at cost containment were tried out. In the 1970s the health maintenance organization (HMO) appeared. It is based on the concept that in the long run patients can be treated more economically if they have easy access to physicians in the incipient stages of disease and if the doctor has a financial incentive to keep an illness from progressing. Under the prepayment plan, a subscriber is assessed a fixed monthly charge, whether he is well or ill. At the first symptom, he is entitled to see one of the physicians in the group that has contracted to provide treatment. All subsequent costs are covered by the prepayment, even if hospitalization or surgery or both are needed. Obviously, it is to the advantage of the physician group to practice preventive medicine. The federal government subsidized some early HMO plans in a study to determine whether the idea was cost effective. The plan was slow in catching on, although in a few communities as much as 20 percent of the population is covered. An HMO that enrolled one-third or one-half of the potential patients in a community would put nonparticipating practitioners at a competitive disadvantage. On the other hand, a group that ventures into an HMO arrangement without reliable actuarial data risks financial ruin if a large number of the subscribers require hospitalization and prolonged treatment. A newer and still largely untried plan is the preferred provider organization (PPO). Basically, it is an arrangement under which a company obtains a preferential rate and treatment for its employees who are covered. A participating group of doctors offers a volume discount to the company in exchange for an expected large influx of patients and immediate payment of bills.

Times had changed, and in 1982 the clinic board of management and the executive committee of the foundation's board of trustees, recognizing this fact, formally adopted a statement entitled "The Mission of the Ochsner Medical Institutions."

> The Ochsner Medical Institutions, based on a highly specialized and skilled multi-specialty group practice, aspire to provide sophisticated patient care of the highest quality to a varied regional and international referral population and to the local population. In fulfilling their role as leaders in health care delivery, the Institutions emphasize the importance of education and research in the support of a comprehensive approach to medical care.
>
> In patient care, education, and research, the Institutions are dedicated to meeting the challenges presented by increasingly complex develop-

ments in medical science and technology and a changing system of delivering medical services. The Institutions are determined to confront these challenges and to remain in the forefront of health care delivery through the continued application and development of medical advancement and innovation, while maintaining economic viability and organizational success.

In *Patient Care*, the Institutions will offer a comprehensive scope of medical services from a variety of practice modalities, ranging from primary care to high level tertiary care, in hospital-based as well as ambulatory arrangements, in an economically feasible manner. The Institutions will continually strive to maintain the level of excellence in medical care necessary to meet the overall needs of their patients and to meet the expectations of the public and the profession.

What the governing councils did overall was to formally spell out the goals and the approaches that were adopted by the management of the institutions in the 1970s and early 1980s as it dealt with the new realities in medicine. Clinic and foundation were prospering, and there was not much need for crisis intervention. Planning was going beyond the do-nothing philosophy noted by Riddick as, "If it ain't broke, don't fix it." The opportunities of the future seemed to lie largely in the practice of primary medicine. "You can't run a big clinic on cancer patients alone," Riddick explained. "There is no such thing, anyway, as a pure tertiary care center." The clinic continues as a medical court of last resort, with highly trained experts in the specialties and subspecialties. But as Riddick puts it, the physicians now double in brass. Ailments to be treated range from acute leukemia to, figuratively, hangnails. The concept gets little argument from the partners. "There has to be relief for the physician," the medical director points out. "One cannot operate on a crisis basis for fifty or sixty hours a week. The doctor would burn out fast if every decision were a life-or-death one, or involved pushing back the frontiers of medical capability. It's nice to see somebody who is nervous and has gas pains. Any practitioner likes to see a tennis elbow once in awhile."

The clinic, explains Riddick, has made a more specific commitment to primary care, acknowledging a need for this type of practice and insisting that the services would not be superficial. "Patients must have access, and there must be coordination among the providers. The interest will be on the whole patient rather than a particular part of the patient." The key doctor at Ochsner in the delivery of primary care is a specialist, the internist, not a general or family practitioner.

But the director knows full well that planning is largely a guessing exercise, for nobody can predict future developments in medicine. He points out that when he finished medical school, planning then based on the state of the art would have assigned a third of his class to long-term psychiatric practice, another third to the treatment of tuberculosis, and a large percentage to taking care of poliomyelitis patients. Now vaccines have almost eliminated polio, drugs control psychiatric problems, and antibiotics deal effectively with tuberculosis. "No plan actually is adhered to for long, because conditions change," Riddick comments. "We're going to look at the environment. We'll keep our eyes open, and take readings."

Hand in hand, foundation and clinic stepped out into activities that had not been pursued before. One idea was the establishment of outposts, satellite clinics. The idea of operating Ochsner satellites was debated by the founders as long ago as 1950. Curtis Tyrone suggested the possibility of opening a branch for obstetrical-gynecological patients in the fast-growing East New Orleans area. The others told him to explore the potential but to proceed in secrecy. Obviously the partners did not want to arouse any more hostility among outside practitioners than already existed. Tyrone's idea died for lack of support.

In 1961 the pinch for space in the ob-gyn department, which was operating in the area of Brent House given over to clinic offices, led to discussions about the desirability of establishing a branch for women patients in the area of Sauve and Hickory roads in Kenner. Guy Caldwell noted after a meeting in February that the board of management "is aware of the fact that this is a policy decision that could open up the possibility of having branch clinics not only in the outlying area of New Orleans, but in outlying areas of Louisiana." A real estate developer offered to construct a building that he would lease to the clinic at $3.60 to $3.70 per square foot per year. Administrator Edgar Saux raised questions about other expenses involved, and the board deferred action. In May, John C. Weed and John B. Holland made a pitch before the staff executive committee for the proposed branch. Two of the young members of the ob-gyn staff, they said, were wasting their time because of the shortage of office space. Weed also noted that New Orleanians were moving out to suburban areas, and Jefferson Parish was growing very rapidly. He predicted that the obstetrical practice could be increased significantly by such a move. The committee favored the branch if additional space could not be provided in Brent House, but the proposal finally died because the completion of the clinic building in 1963 made plenty of office room available.

In 1963 and 1964 the attention of clinic planners turned again to the East New Orleans–Gentilly area, where the Methodist Hospital, now the Pendleton Memorial Methodist Hospital, had recently opened. One of the advocates of establishing a satellite in the neighborhood was neurosurgeon John D. Jackson. But by June 15, 1964, he had second thoughts and wrote in a memorandum to the staff executive committee that the clinic partners should consider carefully before acting. "At the present time," Jackson wrote, "we could not handle the increase in patient load, since the present hospital facilities are already becoming overcrowded. . . . A new branch could not be handled efficiently under the present set-up. We would be placed back in the same situation that we were in when the Clinic Building was next to the Touro Infirmary and the Hospital in Jefferson Parish." Again no action toward setting up a branch clinic was taken.

During this period, a few Ochsner physicians and surgeons were traveling to other cities where specialists in their fields were not well established. Jackson and Homer D. Kirgis, his fellow neurosurgeon, made weekly visits to Gulfport, Mississippi, and Lafayette, Louisiana. Gastroenterologist William A. Ferrante was called on occasion to Alexandria, Louisiana. Orthopedists sometimes were summoned to Hammond, Louisiana. The trips were economically feasible if a doctor could see several patients in a day, and those who needed surgery entered the Ochsner hospital. On the other hand, the board of management came to frown on long journeys for the purpose of attending to a single patient. Alton Ochsner and Dean H. Echols over the years were asked to come to distant states, and even foreign countries, to perform operations. Most specialties now are practiced even in small cities, and there is no longer a demand for clinic staff to make the kind of weekly visits Jackson and Kirgis made to Lafayette and Gulfport, however.

The clinic has always had a strict ban against the participation of its staff in ghost surgery, a practice of some doctors when Ochsner was founded. It was an arrangement under which a practitioner calls in an outside surgeon to do a procedure on a patient that the outsider never meets. The practitioner bills the patient as though he had done the operation himself and splits the fee with the surgeon. The American College of Surgeons and American Medical Association have since eliminated the practice, declaring it to be unethical.

As early as 1956 Dean Echols tried to persuade the founders to set up a branch for the practice of industrial medicine of the type in which an employer contracts with a doctor or group of doctors to provide health services for employees. An arrangement covered preemployment physical examinations, treatment of accident injuries, and often the presence of a physician at an industrial plant to hold sick calls. Echols suggested that the clinic acquire the industrial practice of Dr. Joseph T. Scott, Jr., which he said the year before had a gross income of $150,000 and a net of at least $50,000. Echols predicted the gross could be increased to a million dollars a year, and said the clinic would have an opportunity to build a national reputation by upgrading industrial practice. On February 28, 1956, the partners rejected Echols's proposal. They concluded that industrial medicine was too different from the clinic's usual type of practice and was an activity with which the staff was not familiar. In addition, they feared it would cost $100,000 over a five-year period to implement Echols's ideas and noted the clinic could not then spare the money.

The clinic finally ventured into industrial medicine in 1975 when the board of management brought Francis T. Gidman onto the staff and arranged to continue the services that he had been supplying for the Avondale Shipyards and other plants on the west bank of the Mississippi River. Other clinic partners took over Gidman's duties after his death in 1979.

In an increasingly competitive environment, Ochsner turned to aggressive marketing tactics in order to hold its old patients and attract new ones. Its priceless asset was a reputation for competence and care won over a forty-year span. The first concerns of Porter and Riddick were to nurture the staff that had made the name and to maintain the physical plant in which that staff could practice effectively. They also had to bring in the patients to support the institutions. Their opportunities lay in supplying the services demanded by the public and in promoting and making them known.

The founders would have applauded the marketing strategy. They promoted the clinic and foundation hospital and went after patients as openly as the medical customs of their day permitted. However, there were strictures that limited the amount of publicity jealous rivals would tolerate, and Alton Ochsner and his associates tried not to cross the line. On the few occasions when the Orleans Parish Medical Society reported complaints by other members, the partners took pains to appease the complainants. The attempt to keep doctors out of the public eye was a hangover from times when medicine was an arcane science and the public gullible. By the 1970s professional attitudes became more liberal. Medical centers maintain public relations departments that have the duty of spreading the word about services offered and the accomplishments of the staff. Ochsner's promotions stay within the precedents set by other institutions and accepted by the profession.

The founders themselves had a part of the clinic's first marketing project aimed at bringing in a flow of patients who needed only primary care. In 1954 they joined in the decision to establish an executive health program, in which as many as five hundred business firms have been involved at a time. Most of the participating companies pay the fees for annual checkups for executives and key employees, who get a one-day screening designed to uncover potential health problems or a more elaborate two-day going over. For three decades executive health not only has contributed to the work load for internists and laboratories but also has persuaded the men and women who have undergone checkups and members of their families to come to Ochsner when they need medical attention.

The proliferation of on-campus activities began in 1976 with the opening of a fitness center, or health club, in the newly expanded Brent House. It is equipped with the paraphernalia for supervised body-building exercises and manned by physical-training experts. Participants include staff doctors as well as patients, and a special routine is offered for the rehabilitation of victims of heart attacks. In the same year came the beginning of the antismoking clinic, an outgrowth of Alton Ochsner's prolonged campaign against cigarettes. Psychologist Robert P. Baker devised a program employing psychological methods for helping patients overcome the smoking habit. One ploy, the aversion technique, is to confine a smoker in a tiny room until he gags from the fumes of numerous burning cigarettes.

Measures aimed at attracting primary care patients gained momentum in 1979 with the creation of a section of preventive medicine, also known as prospective medicine, in the department of medicine. Internist Brooks Emory was chosen as first head of the section of physicians who try to keep a patient well by assessing his physical condition and evaluating risk factors and prescribing regimens to ward off illnesses. In the same year a weight control clinic came into being. Dieticians, exercise physiologists, and psychologists provide a program of behavior modification, physical exercise, and aversion conditioning to assist patients in losing pounds.

Four other activities took form in 1981, a banner year for partners who want the clinic to become more involved in primary care. Neurologist Jeffrey P. Ellison took charge of a stroke center, which has the purpose of preventing strokes. When early warnings such as transitory loss of vision or numbness are recognized, aggressive treatment can sometimes head off a stroke. A stress treatment unit was organized to teach stress management skills to adults and older adolescents with stress-related illnesses. The patients learn to deal with headaches, backaches, sleeplessness, and other psychosomatic problems. Albert Segaloff, veteran researcher in breast cancer, and William McKinnon were placed in command of a breast-screening center. Those who come to the clinic are given diagnostic tests and taught to make self-examinations. Paul Jorgenson, former assistant trainer for the New Orleans Saints professional football team, joined the staff of the division of sports medicine, a section of the orthopedics department. Treatment is offered to persons who are injured in athletic activities, and full coverage provided for high school players.

Perhaps the most significant of the on-campus innovations is the Ochsner Community Internal Medicine Section, created in 1982 and directed by Michael C. Tooke. Ten internists provide twenty-four-hour coverage in a program to make Ochsner services quickly accessible to residents of the metropolitan area. The section has its own telephone number, and callers are assured of getting attention expeditiously, without awaiting their turns for appointments in the regular clinic ro-

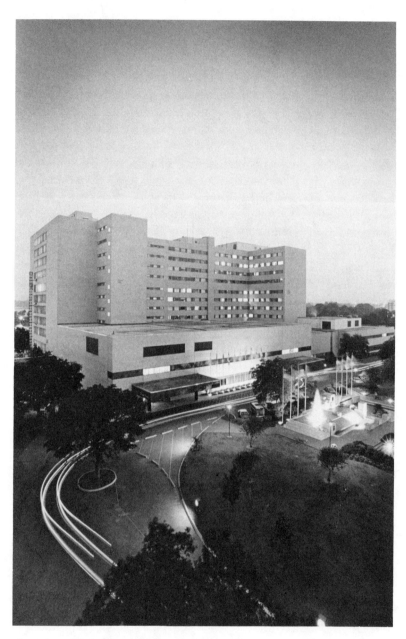

The Ochsner Medical Institutions today

tation. Section members treat problems that do not require the laboratory and X-ray procedures that are available for the seriously ill or those with complaints that are difficult to diagnose. The section does not duplicate the activities of the acute medicine physicians or those of the hospital emergency room staff. Tooke and his associates are primary care specialists.

Once this array of services was functioning, the clinic and foundation reached out for people to patronize them. "The Ochsner Wellness Series" was advertised in such publications as *Time*, *Newsweek*, *Sports Illustrated*, and *U.S. News & World Report* and over local radio stations. "You have a choice, you know," the public was told. "You can improve the quality of your life right now with these proven, no-nonsense programs at Ochsner. Health Appraisal. Stress Management. Weight Control. Smoking Elimination. Fitness Center."

The responsibility for making the public aware of Ochsner's expanding services, for cementing the involvement of supporters in the institutions' activities, and for fund raising fell upon Thomas P. Gore, who was brought to the foundation as director of public affairs and later promoted to the post of vice president, public affairs and resource development. Gore's know-how resulted in widespread coverage of Ochsner accomplishments and human interest events in newspapers, television, and radio. He instituted radio and television programs featuring Ochsner doctors who offered listeners advice on how to stay well. Foundation publications, *Inside Ochsner* and *Ochsner Reports*, got a typographical facelift and progressed beyond routine company publication coverage into articles that won general readership. In a coup without precedent Gore arranged for *Ochsner Reports* to be printed quarterly as advertising matter in the *Times-Picayune*'s *Dixie Magazine*, thereby increasing the circulation twentyfold. The publications brought national awards for excellence.

It was not only on-campus that Ochsner branched out. After the years of discussion, the first and then the second of the clinic's outposts were opened, and the industrial medicine practice begun in 1978 was broadened into a department of occupational medicine. The institutions set out to become the medical sentinel for the Port of New Orleans and for the industrial complex that stretches along both sides of the Mississippi River from New Orleans to Baton Rouge. The clinic also set up an offshoot professional corporation to staff a state hospital seventy-five miles away.

"Little Ochsner" is the nickname some Houma residents bestowed on the state's charity hospital there—the 175-bed South Louisiana Medical Center. The family resemblance is not striking, but there is a connection. Ochsner interns and residents make up the house staff, and the professional staff is an adjunct of the clinic.

The arrangement came about because of the need for additional training opportunities for Ochsner's fellows, all 210 of whom cannot receive enough exposure to patients in the Ochsner Foundation Hospital alone. At the time, the state of Louisiana was casting about for doctors to man the new Houma hospital when it opened in 1978. In the fifties, sixties, and into the seventies, Ochsner surgical fellows had rotated in staffing the E. A. Conway Charity Hospital in Monroe, Louisiana. The Louisiana State University Medical School at Shreveport gradually put its graduates into house staff positions there, however, and the surgical program was a burden to Ochsner partners who took turns making the two-hundred-mile flight to Monroe to supervise the fellows. Completion of the Houma hospital finally offered an opportunity of training more interns and residents in a facility only seventy-five miles from the campus.

State officials also talked with Frank Riddick about having the Ochsner Clinic provide the senior staff, as well. Ochsner declined, but a compromise was arranged. Riddick and other partners borrowed $100,000 from the clinic and formed a professional corporation, the South Louisiana Medical Associates. They hired a staff, now grown to thirty doctors, which runs the medical services. A problem was the limit on doctors' salaries imposed by state civil service. It was solved because the Houma hospital is permitted to accept private patients when beds are available. Many patients have Medicare or Medicaid or insurance coverage and the income from this source is used to supplement state pay. The SLMA began offering its services on September 18, 1978, and it is now financially in the clear. Riddick is president of the associates, who have no formal affiliation with the clinic. Clinic doctors who supervise the fellows travel between the campus and Houma in a passenger van, which makes two daily round trips.

It came as no surprise, in view of Ochsner's experience, when some

Houma practitioners condemned the arrangement and accused the clinic of stealing patients. At a meeting of the medical society in Houma, Riddick pointed out that state officials had attempted without success to interest Houma doctors in staffing the hospital. He offered to pull the South Louisiana Medical Associates out of the facility if the local practitioners would take over. Merrill O. Hines recalled that he had come under fire from physicians at Monroe while Ochsner was involved in the training program at E. A. Conway.

The clinic's first outpost, the Houma/Bayou Area Dialysis Center, was built in 1978 and began its activities in November of that year. Internist Charles M. Kantrow, director of the facility, supervised the planning and construction of the red-brick structure on a one-acre tract near the South Louisiana Medical Center on the outskirts of Houma. The clinic invested $120,000 to obtain the land and finance and equip the building. As many as forty-two patients can be treated in the facility. In thrice-weekly four-hour sessions, the blood of patients who have lost kidney function is purified by being circulated through artificial kidneys. Most of the cost is borne by government programs.

The second outpost, the Ochsner Clinic Riverfront Occupational Medicine and Environmental Health Center, was first housed in the New Orleans General Hospital, formerly Sara Mayo, at 625 Jackson Avenue, in the waterfront district, and later moved to the clinic building. The center became an Ochsner facility in 1982 with the addition of Velma L. Campbell to the staff. Victor Alexander, who became head of the occupational medicine department, said the riverfront center would "care for patients with occupational illnesses and injuries, operate medical surveillance programs on contract, perform preemployment and annual physicals, provide consultation services to unions, industry and government agencies, and conduct medical evaluations for environmental health problems."

Alexander came to the clinic in 1982 from the federal Occupational Safety and Health Administration, which he had joined as its first staff physician. Although he has since retired, his department continues to offer employee health services to the operators of industrial plants and guides them in protecting the environment and in work safety measures. Alexander saw Ochsner's involvement as a logical followup to the long crusade that Alton Ochsner conducted against smoking—

"the free-spirited, intellectual approach," he called it. Alexander was one of Ochsner's spokesmen in discussions with industrialists about a program based on the preferred provider organization concept. He noted that with a big staff of specialists and up-to-date facilities for ambulatory care, Ochsner could offer cost-effective treatment, helping companies to control their health-related expenses. Most PPO-type plans provide for a review of charges that the subscriber wants to challenge. In 1983 Ochsner tiptoed into the still-experimental area of preferred provider organizations. A department was set up to deal with firms or organizations that were interested in the concept, and the first contract for applying the plan was signed shortly before the end of the year with the Jefferson Parish Sheriff's Department. Only the experience of months or years would decide whether the PPO would become an important part of Ochsner activities. Certainly, the occupational medicine department is counted on to help Ochsner keep its share of patients.

Not long after the first PPO contract was signed, Ochsner stepped into the realm of health maintenance organizations, hiring a director to organize one of the first HMO operations in New Orleans. Management expected that in the foreseeable future most of the clinic's practice would continue on a fee-for-service basis but projected that thousands of patients would be covered by the prepayment plan. In early 1984 a marketing department was created to spearhead the efforts to promote the care offered by clinic and hospital.

After some thirty-five years of intermittent discussion, the clinic in 1984 arranged to open its first true satellites in 1985. One will be in Marrero, on the west bank of the Mississippi River, and the other in Kenner, on the east bank. The board of management had decided to put doctors where the patients are instead of waiting for those needing treatment to find their way to the clinic. The program called for each satellite to be staffed by internists, pediatricians, and obstetricians practicing primary medicine. Each facility was to have X-ray and basic laboratory equipment. Patients needing specialized treatment were to be sent to the main clinic. Satellites in other locations in the New Orleans area are planned.

A satellite of a sort had already been established. The Ochsner Clinic was selected over seven other bidders to provide on-site medical services at the Louisiana World Exposition, which opened in 1984 on the Mississippi riverfront near Canal Street. Riddick arranged to have a team of physicians, nurses, and technicians on the grounds to provide emergency care of illnesses and injuries. Richard Y. McConnell, head of the department of emergency medicine, was put in charge of the mini clinic. The fair management provided space for Ochsner to present an exhibit on medical advances.

McConnell also became medical director for the New Orleans Aviation Board and, as such, responsible for medical services at the New Orleans International Airport. His task is to arrange for emergency treatment of passengers arriving at and departing from the airport and to direct medical activities in the event of a plane crash. In a disaster, personnel from the Ochsner Medical Institutions are to be flown to the scene in helicopters.

As the Louisiana Power and Light Company neared the completion of the only nuclear plant in the area at Taft, on the west bank of the Mississippi about twenty miles above the hospital, the Ochsner center was chosen as the facility to which employees of the Waterford III plant would be taken in the event of an accident or of exposure to radiation.

Although many of the day-by-day developments in the late 1970s and early 1980s were concerned with bringing patients needing primary care to Ochsner, management never forgot the institutions' commitment to the seriously ill, those requiring the attention of experts with specialized skills. The 1982 statement of mission reiterated that part of Ochsner's reason for being is the provision of high-level tertiary services. It is, of course, a reaffirmation of the original purpose of the founders.

With his background in cancer research, George Porter encouraged the establishment in the fall of 1981 of the Ochsner Cancer Institute, a joint project of foundation and clinic. Several months after becoming president of the foundation, Porter had initiated the Ochsner Cancer Fund and provided a gift of seed money in the names of his parents, Sallie Mapp and George H. Porter, Jr. Riddick joined him in announcing the creation of the institute, devoted to treatment, education, research, and the development of a major cancer referral center at Ochsner. Pathologist Gist H. Farr, Jr., the first director, spent a year getting the institute organized, then turned over the reins to colon and rectal surgeon Bernard T. Ferrari. The institute operates a computerized tumor registry that provides detailed information on all Ochsner cancer patients. It shares information with other cancer centers, enabling Ferrari's aides to furnish clinic physicians and surgeons with up-to-date data on the results of various methods of treatment of the different types of cancer. "We'll try to influence our doctors and help them do a better job," Ferrari explains. The institute is involved in patient-support services, including education, home care, and the adjustment of families to the needs of cancer victims. The activity is liberally supported by the clinic and foundation but depends also on public contributions. Ferrari has centered his appeal for funds on suburban business and professional sources. He also seeks governmental aid.

Looking to the future, the clinic board of management voted late in 1982 to appropriate a fund to reward staff members who carry on innovative research aimed at developing new methods of treatment and attracting first-time patients. The action, strongly supported by Riddick, in effect provides what is known in business as R and D, research and development, money. It finances a core laboratory, manned by scientists, to work with practitioners who experiment with new procedures in their specialties. The board recognized that a staff doctor who spends hours in a laboratory is contributing as much to the welfare of the clinic as is a colleague who is seeing patients all day long. Staff income is based largely on production—the billing of patients. Thus, the creation of the fund allows the board to give credit for research and prevents a partner from losing money while he is experimenting. A subcommittee that included William Ferrante, Edward Genton, and Richard Ré recommended that the laboratory be involved originally in work in molecular biology and bend its efforts to the support of clinically relevant collaborative research. "The uniqueness provided by medical excellence hinges not only on adequate amenities for patients and state-of-the-art health care, but also on *innovative therapy and diagnosis*," the subcommittee commented.

What amounted to a vote of confidence in management strategies came in 1983 when the clinic partners agreed to resume the annual donations to the foundation that had been suspended in 1978 when the enlargement of the clinic building resulted in a much higher rent paid to the landlord foundation. The 1983 contribution of $600,000, which bolstered the research program, was an investment in the institutions' future. Each partner's portion of the gift was substantial; the staff doctors were following the lead of earlier generations in shouldering a hefty part of the burden.

Jeanie

Jeanie of the dark blue eyes. Jeanie the indestructible. Jeanie, one in nearly a million, but special. Very special.

A quarter of a century after Ochsner Clinic practitioners used their surgical and medical arts to open up a bright future for the Mouton Siamese twins, Jeanie came along to prove that the magic still works.

A picture remains frozen in the minds of those who saw her—Jeanie Marie Thibodeaux—in the pediatric intensive care unit at the Ochsner Foundation Hospital. There she was, sitting upright in her crib, watching with lively curiosity the activity going on around her. No tears, no moans, no fretting suggested that only twenty-four hours earlier she had undergone the ordeal of open-heart surgery. There was evidence enough. Long tubes connected her tiny body to life-sustaining equipment along the wall. A fresh incision stretching halfway around her torso almost connected with the fading scar of another that reached the rest of the way around. No whining or plea for sympathy came when her mother, Mrs. Joseph O. Thibodeaux, and then her father picked her up and sat in a chair beside the crib, gently rocking her so as not to disconnect the tubes.

At fifteen months of age, Jeanie had learned to deal with pain and the threat of death. Seven times already she had received the last rites of the Roman Catholic church. Twice she had been flown in an ambulance plane to the hospital. On two other occasions she had been brought in a surface ambulance, and twice more she had made the trip in her parents' automobile.

She was only four hours old when she made the first ambulance flight, from Opelousas, Louisiana, where she was born on July 20, 1979. One problem was a tracheo-esophageal fistula, a gap in the esophagus that caused reflux from the stomach to flow into the trachea and the lungs. This resulted in recurrent attacks of pneumonia.

Several times she was barely revived with mouth-to-mouth resuscitation. Dr. Charles C. Bertrand, who referred her to Ochsner, saw her through one crisis after another.

At Ochsner she came under the care of Robert M. Arensman, pediatric surgeon, who worked out the procedures that would save Jeanie with all the care that Alton Ochsner had given to the separation of Catherine and Carolyn Mouton. First, as soon as Jeanie could withstand the operation, Arensman repaired the esophagus. But the reflux continued, as did the pneumonia. The next operation was a Nissen fundolication in which the surgeon utilized a part of Jeanie's stomach to create a flutter valve that finally slowed the reflux. Jeanie's troubles still were not over. She also was afflicted with patent ductus arteriosus, a condition in which a fetal blood vessel fails to close at birth. The repair of this anomaly was the open-heart surgery from which Jeanie was recovering so amazingly when she showed her spunk in the intensive care unit that afternoon in October, 1980. Afterwards, her parents brought her by car from their home in St. Landry, Louisiana, for occasional checkups at Ochsner. At three, her weight of thirty-two pounds, a good average, showed that she had caught up with other children of her age group. She still has occasional spells of pneumonia, but Arensman and Bertrand are hopeful that she will outgrow the problem.

Jeanie is No. 636062 in a roll of clinic patients that before long will reach the million mark, one of many in a vast horde of men, women, and children who came for help to the institutions created long ago by the five professors. Her case is submerged in a sea of numbers, but Alton Ochsner, Guy Caldwell, Edgar Burns, Duke LeJeune, and Curtis Tyrone would have taken a special pride in the treatment that she received and in the promising results. In Jeanie there is a demonstration that their successors have not lost the dedication and the skills that made the institutions what they are, that bode so well for the future.

Index